Developing Military Health Care Leaders

Insights from the Military, Civilian, and Government Sectors

Sheila Nataraj Kirby, Julie A. Marsh, Jennifer Sloan McCombs,

Harry J. Thie, Nailing Xia, Jerry M. Sollinger

Prepared for the Office of the Secretary of Defense

Approved for public release; distribution unlimited

Center for Military Health Policy Research

A JOINT ENDEAVOR OF RAND HEALTH AND THE
RAND NATIONAL DEFENSE RESEARCH INSTITUTE

The research reported here was sponsored by the Office of the Secretary of Defense (OSD). The research was conducted jointly by the Center for Military Health Policy Research, a RAND Health program, and the Forces and Resources Policy Center, a RAND National Defense Research Institute (NDRI) program. NDRI is a federally funded research and development center sponsored by OSD, the Joint Staff, the Unified Combatant Commands, the Navy, the Marine Corps, the defense agencies, and the defense Intelligence Community under Contract W74V8H-06-C-0002.

Library of Congress Control Number: 2011920369

ISBN: 978-0-8330-5007-6

Published 2011 by the RAND Corporation
1776 Main Street, P.O. Box 2138, Santa Monica, CA 90407-2138
1200 South Hayes Street, Arlington, VA 22202-5050
4570 Fifth Avenue, Suite 600, Pittsburgh, PA 15213-2665
RAND URL: http://www.rand.org/
To order RAND documents or to obtain additional information, contact
Distribution Services: Telephone: (310) 451-7002;
Fax: (310) 451-6915; Email: order@rand.org

Preface

The U.S. military has been at war for nearly a decade, and the long-running conflicts have placed enormous stress on the Military Health System (MHS). These operations, coupled with rising health care costs and the need to operate easily in joint environments, have caused military health leaders to recognize the need to transform the MHS. The 2006 Quadrennial Defense Review highlighted the importance of preparing health care leaders to succeed in joint, performance-based environments. As part of a larger project providing assistance to the MHS in establishing a joint medical education and training campus at Fort Sam Houston, Texas, the RAND Corporation was asked to examine the ways in which leaders in the medical field are prepared and supported in the civilian and military sectors, to review the competencies necessary to be a leader in the current environment, and to recommend improvements to the ways in which potential leaders are identified and developed for leadership positions in the MHS.

This research was sponsored the MHS Office of Transformation and conducted jointly by RAND Health's Center for Military Health Policy Research and the Forces and Resources Policy Center of the RAND National Defense Research Institute (NDRI). The Center for Military Health Policy Research taps RAND expertise in both defense and health policy to conduct research for the Department of Defense, the Veterans Administration, and nonprofit organizations. RAND Health aims to transform the well-being of all people by solving complex problems in health and health care. NDRI is a federally funded research and development center sponsored by the Office of the Secretary of Defense, the Joint Staff, the Unified Combatant Commands, the Navy, the Marine Corps, the defense agencies, and the defense Intelligence Community.

For more information on the Center for Military Health Policy Research, see http://www.rand.org/multi/military/ or contact the co-directors (contact information is provided on the web page). For more information on the Forces and Resources Policy Center, see http://www.rand.org/nsrd/about/frp.html or contact the director (contact information is provided on the web page).

Contents

Figures

Tables

Summary

Background and Purpose

Over the past few years, military leaders have realized that the Military Health System (MHS) has to transform itself and the way it does business. This need has been driven by the rapid escalation in the costs of health care, a changing environment with an increased emphasis on performance management, the unprecedented challenges facing the U.S. military at home and abroad that require it to assume new roles and responsibilities, and the need to transform the medical force so that future medical support is fully aligned with joint force concepts. As part of a larger project providing assistance to the MHS in establishing a joint medical education and training campus at Fort Sam Houston, Texas, RAND was asked to examine the ways in which leaders in the health care field are prepared and supported in the civilian and military sectors, to review the competencies necessary to be a leader in the current environment, and to recommend improvements to the ways in which potential leaders are identified and developed for leadership positions in the MHS.[1]

A primary goal of officer management is to produce qualified senior leaders who can function in both joint and service-specific environments and who have the competencies that are important for successful leadership. Our framework assumes that military medical officers are functionally qualified and continue to develop their domain knowledge and skills. Thus, our focus is on who is developed and where and how these officers receive the knowledge, experience, and acculturation necessary to qualify them for leadership in both service and joint environments. An organization's approach to leader development plays out against the larger backdrop of the local, regional, national, and global context, which shapes what an organization expects from leaders and how it designs and implements development strategies. These contextual factors also enable or constrain the ability of an organization to develop the needed leaders. There are three important dimensions of an organization's approach to leader development: how it

---

[1] We use the term *leader* to identify an individual who is likely to be in a command or executive position in an organization.

selects individuals who have the potential to be leaders, how it develops them, and how it incentivizes them to apply for and remain in leadership positions.

Data and Methods

The study encompassed several tasks, including a review of the literature on leader development and the creation of a conceptual framework to guide data collection and analysis. The conceptual framework focused on how organizations select "high-potentials" for leader development, the strategies that organizations use to incentivize and develop these leaders, and the extent to which the overall approach is systematic and purposeful. Obviously, an organization's approach to leader development is affected by the context and the organizational environment and guided by explicit and implicit expectations for leaders. Using this framework as the basis for our interview protocol, we conducted structured interviews with 57 military health professions officers[2] and community managers and with 30 civilian health care leaders in 25 organizations. We also conducted a case study of how one government agency—the Veterans Health Administration (VHA)—approaches executive leader development. The case study included interviews with 16 top-level leaders and network and facility directors. The interviews were conducted over a period of two years—2007 through 2009. The MHS, the VHA, and the civilian health care organizations examined in this study are all facing the same kinds of pressures with respect to delivering high-quality health care while struggling with escalating costs and rising demand. As a result, lessons learned by the VHA and civilian health care organizations about designing and implementing leader development policies may have considerable relevance for the military.

Findings

Data from these interviews, along with our extensive review of service documents and the literature on the subject, provide a rich portrait of how health care leaders are currently developed in the three sectors, the competencies necessary to be a successful leader in today's environment, perceived gaps in leader development, and some perceived best practices.

---

[2]   Following U.S. Department of Defense (DoD) Directive 6000.12 (1996), we use the term *health professions officers* when referring to officers who are "serving in the Medical Corps, the Dental Corps, the Veterinary Corps, the Nurse Corps, the Medical Service Corps, the Army Medical Specialist Corps, the Biomedical Sciences Corps, officers whom the Secretaries of the Military Departments have designated as 'qualified in specified healthcare functions,' and those members in DoD programs leading to commissioning in, assignment to, or designation for service in any of those Corps" (Enclosure 2). When referring more generally to leaders in the civilian and military sectors, and in the Veterans Health Administration (VHA) more generally, we use the term *health care leaders*.

Our findings are organized around four research topics:

- desired attributes of leaders in the health care field
- military officers' perceptions about how well the current system works in preparing health professions officers to lead and succeed in performance-based and joint environments
- lessons learned from civilian health care organizations and the VHA regarding leader development
- recommendations to improve leader development of health professions officers in the services.

Desired Attributes of Health Care Leaders

To determine the kinds of knowledge, skills, and experience that organizations believe that leaders need, we reviewed a number of civilian health care leadership competency frameworks, the High Performance Development Model adopted by the VHA, and the military health care leadership competencies identified by the Joint Medical Executive Skills Program (JMESP) as necessary for successful command of a medical treatment facility or for other executive MHS positions. In addition, we asked respondents about the attributes that organizations looked for in their senior leaders—the skills, knowledge, attitudes, and experiences that organizations expected of their executives. Perhaps not surprisingly, there was remarkable consistency in the set of competencies identified both by the frameworks and individuals, which we categorized into three types of competencies and experiences.

First, *management knowledge and experience* includes the skills and abilities to effectively manage financial, human, and information resources to ensure successful fulfillment of organizational goals. Respondents often described the need for both "hard" and "soft" skills. Identified common hard-skill competencies that fall into this category include human resource (HR) management (such as recruitment, staffing, training, and evaluation and assessment), financial resource management (such as budgeting, asset management, and monitoring of financial resources), and information and technology management. The soft skills, or interpersonal and communication skills (with internal and external customers), were considered equally important.

Second, *leadership knowledge and experience* provides strategic and visionary guidance to help the organization meet future challenges. Competencies that fall into this category include visionary leadership (i.e., envisioning a future state and influencing movement toward it), change leadership (i.e., continuously seeking innovative approaches and welcoming changes as opportunities for improvement), flexibility and adaptability, and creative and strategic thinking and planning.

Third, *enterprise knowledge and experience* includes competencies that demonstrate a sound understanding of the profession and the organization, such as organizational awareness or stewardship; an understanding of the larger context in which the organization operates (or systems-level thinking); and an understanding of the global environment.

All our respondents stressed the importance of educational achievement and competency in functional areas. In addition, several respondents also emphasized the importance of leaders who possess strong values and moral character ("a strong moral compass") in addition to knowledge, skills, and abilities. According to several civilian and VHA respondents, a strong values orientation (e.g., organizational stewardship, integrity, financial responsibility) is included in competency profiles for top executives. Diversity of experience, practice in both managing and leading, and, in some cases, an understanding of and experience with the higher levels of the organization were mentioned as critical for leaders.

Respondents were divided in terms of the extent to which health care leaders should possess and maintain clinical skills. Some physician respondents—both military and civilian—stated that the greatest credibility of a health care leader comes from being a physician. In keeping with this belief, the Air Force has a policy of reserving command of medical centers and hospitals for physicians (Medical Corps, or MC). In contrast, the Army and the Navy have opened up these positions to all corps. Military respondents referred to these diametrically opposed policies as "best in breed" versus "best in show." Most respondents (including some Air Force leaders) felt that the Air Force policy was shortsighted and out of step with practice in the civilian sector and organizations like the VHA, in which hospital leaders are often not physicians. Several leaders noted that clinical skills do not automatically translate into leadership skills.

Military Respondents' Perceptions of the Current System of Leader Development

Context, Organizational Environment, and Organizational Leader Expectations. Several respondents recognized the complexity of the military environment and its effects on leader expectations. Particularly among Army and Navy respondents, leaders noted that the military and their respective services had become quite complex on a number of levels: for example, challenges of managing a workforce that now includes military, civilian, and contract workers; dealing with the stresses and demands of war and the disruptions caused by deployments; and new productivity demands and attention to the "bottom line." All shape what is expected of leaders and how they are selected and evaluated.

Respondents in all three services identified differences in opportunities for leadership and growth across the corps. Several leaders in the Army and Navy believed that, when compared to Medical Service Corps (MSC) officers (who are trained in medical administration and other nonclinical skills), MC officers (who are doctors) are at a disadvantage in acquiring leadership skills. Some respondents believed that, given the length of time required for clinical training and the demand to keep officers in clinical positions, it often takes longer and is more difficult for MC providers to gain the requisite skills, although they have greater opportunities to move into leadership positions.

Some Navy respondents criticized the Navy's "lock-step" requirement that an individual must be a director, then an executive officer, then a commanding officer, pointing out that this system overlooks other opportunities for individuals to develop or demonstrate leadership skills. Some respondents noted that rank does not equate to leadership and that physicians, in particular, were often placed in leadership positions because of rank without the requisite experience and training.

Although some respondents in all three services were aware of a set of formal leadership competencies endorsed by the military, most did not remember the name (JMESP), and few found them to be particularly meaningful or consequential.

Overall Approach to Leader Development. There was variation across and within the services in terms of respondents' perceptions of how purposeful and systematic the services are in developing leaders. Most Air Force respondents considered the Air Force to have a reasonable and well-defined system in place for leader development and mentioned both the flight paths and the development teams as the formal process for managing careers. Perceptions were more mixed in the other two services, with some respondents characterizing the approach as lacking purposeful planning and design; they used descriptions such as "happenstance," "serendipity," and "being in the right place at the right time."

How to Select. All services use formal and informal methods to select high-potentials, but perceptions about the efficacy of these approaches varied. Most respondents in all three services viewed formal evaluation reports as one of the primary methods for identifying individuals with leadership potential, with below-the-zone promotions and "getting ranked" as important indicators of high leadership potential. Nevertheless, there was widespread concern about the limitations of these reports, including inflated ratings, subjectivity, the use of "code words" as discriminators, a lack of writing skills on the part of the raters, and raters being too far removed in rank from those being evaluated. Many respondents also mentioned the role that boards play in identifying and selecting individuals for leadership positions and leader development, but some expressed concern about the "soundness" and objectivity of this process. A few respondents mentioned interviews as another formal and effective way to select leaders, but this approach did not seem to be widely used. Many respondents across the services noted that an "informal system" with information gleaned from colleagues and word of mouth greatly affected the identification of leaders and potential leaders, and that these were often more important than formal methods in selecting leaders at the highest levels.

While a few were satisfied with the timing of selection for leadership opportunities and training, several leaders in the Army and Navy argued that identification needed to occur earlier than it currently does. For example, many Navy leaders believed that formal development opportunities often came too late in one's career to be useful and that the Navy needs to be more proactive in providing opportunities to individuals before they are in leadership positions, rather than offering them "after the fact, when you take over one of these organizations." As discussed earlier, in all three services, respondents mentioned that physicians do not receive leader development opportunities early enough in their careers and often lack leadership and management skills and experience. Some respondents, particularly those in the Navy, mentioned the need to accord diversity more consideration in the selection process.

How to Develop. In our interviews, approaches to developing high-potential candidates as described by respondents fell into three broad categories: job assignments, education and training, and mentoring.

Job Assignments. Many of our respondents viewed on-the-job experience as the most valuable and effective means of developing leaders, but not all were satisfied with this emphasis. Others felt that this approach was particularly challenging for physicians. Most agreed that diversity of job experience and wide exposure to different types of jobs and responsibilities are important for leader development.

Enterprise knowledge and experience are increasingly seen as important for military leaders as operations become more joint and integrated (i.e., interservice, interagency, intergovernmental, and multinational). Across the services, many respondents considered joint experiences to be beneficial to leader development; however, they did not tend to endorse mandatory requirements for joint experience and assignments, noting that the lack of joint billets available to health care officers made mandating them difficult.

Education and Training. Almost all our respondents described receiving formal education and training for certain positions and commands. However, views were mixed about the value of the current education and training. Some believed that certain courses were valuable; others noted that coursework must be teamed with experiential learning. Leaders across the services cited a need for better writing skills and more instruction on the business aspects of medicine, particularly for clinicians.

All respondents discussed senior-level professional military education opportunities, including their service's war college and the National War College. Almost all agreed that in-residence attendance at war college was far more valuable than completing the coursework through correspondence, which was viewed as a way of merely "checking a box." However, several leaders noted downsides to resident participation, including the high opportunity costs for both the individual and the service. Navy respondents were more critical of that service's war college in terms of the time needed to complete the coursework, the limited slots available, the potential for doctors to lose their bonuses, and the lack of planning in subsequent career assignments that prevented some physicians from applying what they learned.

Respondents were hesitant to endorse mandatory joint education, given the limited number of seats at schools offering joint professional military education.

Respondents across the services identified the value of educational and training opportunities provided by individuals and organizations outside of the military, many of which are sponsored by the services. These included graduate school, strategic leadership courses, and the Interagency Institute for Federal Health Care Executives. In other cases, leaders across the services described seeking out their own education outside of the military (such as courses offered by the American College of Healthcare Executives).

Mentoring. There was widespread agreement across the services that mentoring was important for leader development, and almost all respondents described personal experiences with mentoring or being mentored. Mentor relationships were initiated from either the top or the bottom. While some leaders noted that their service had a formal mentoring system, almost all described informal mentoring and tended to believe that it was more effective than formal mentoring programs.

How to Incentivize. Several respondents described how leaders were motivated to participate in certain "development opportunities" because they greatly affect promotion and command opportunities (for example, the advanced professional military education courses). Others related their own decision to seek education and assignments to promotion incentives. Several respondents mentioned that retention was an important constraining factor in the ability to identify, grow, and mentor high-potentials and that the military needed to look at ways to retain good people. In particular, some respondents mentioned that two-year assignments were short and disruptive to families and acted as a disincentive to retention.

Lessons Learned from Civilian Health Care Organizations and the VHA Regarding Leader Development

Our interviews with leaders in civilian health care organizations and the VHA mirrored research findings about best practices in leader development and also provided some additional insights. Next, we highlight some practices that leaders in these organizations believed were important or effective.

Context, Organizational Environment, and Organizational Leader Expectations. Two major themes emerged in this area. One was the importance of supporting leadership development at the highest level and the belief that "investing in leadership is as or more important than other investments and priorities." This includes investing in infrastructure resources and making a commitment to managing the process of identifying potential leaders. A second was the need to develop a "living" competency model that is linked to organizational goals and strategic improvement plans—a model that drives the organization's approach to leader development. In these organizations, the leader's competencies were infused throughout the leader development process, guiding recruitment and selection, assessment of needs for professional and management development, development of programs, and evaluation.

Approach to Leader Development. Most organizations adopted purposeful approaches that were clearly aligned with the strategic and business goals of the organization.

How to Select. In addition to succession planning, respondents reported that their organizations were thoughtful and deliberate in their recruiting, interviewing, and hiring processes for executives. Several respondents reported using behavioral interview questions to identify individuals who possessed the competencies and behaviors they sought, while others mentioned specific screening techniques to assess individuals' values. The U.S. Department of Veterans Affairs uses performance-based interviewing extensively as a selection and assessment tool. Some civilian and VHA respondents mentioned that it was important to develop not only people with high potential but also "solid performers" because they are the "bread and butter" of the organization and also need opportunities for growth.

Several respondents considered diversity issues when deciding whom to target. One organization felt strongly that it needed to be proactive to better ensure that the hospital staff reflected the community. Respondents from civilian organizations described diversity strategies aimed at ensuring that more women and minorities were promoted to senior roles, which involved working to develop these candidates at less senior levels.

How to Develop. Respondents mentioned that their leader development programs went beyond the traditional classroom format to include some or all of the following: stretch assignments or details to leader positions, short-term projects overseen by preceptors, 360-degree or other rigorous types of assessment and feedback, mentoring or coaching, personal development plans, and structured reflection. Promising specific strategies included the following:

- job assignments
- coaching or mentoring
- cross-functional and team development
- 360-degree feedback.

Respondents also stressed the need to evaluate these strategies on a regular basis and to revise or adapt them as needed to improve their effectiveness.

How to Incentivize. Respondents from both civilian organizations in our sample and the VHA reported involving top executives in some form of annual performance-based evaluation. These processes tend to emphasize evaluation based on measurable metrics that are tied to broader organizational goals as well as to individual ones, and they generally link to incentive or compensation plans based on weighted formulas. Some organizations seem to focus exclusively on outcomes and measurable objectives. While most systems evaluate what leaders accomplish over the year, some also assess how they have accomplished their goals. The "how" tends to be guided by leadership competencies and was described by some as the "non-measurables," such as how an individual develops others, handles HR issues, and demonstrates organizational stewardship, among other things. A handful of respondents noted the importance of nonpecuniary rewards and recognition for leaders and emerging leaders. These approaches could include providing a special title or project to individuals with demonstrated talent or accomplishments.

Recommendations

Overall, the majority of our military respondents believed, with some caveats, that the services do a good job of preparing their military health care leaders for executive positions in the MHS by using a multipronged approach that includes job assignments, education and training, informal mentoring, and annual reviews. Their comments, along with those of our civilian and VHA respondents, suggest possible avenues for change and improvement. To distill lessons learned about effective ways to develop leaders for executive positions, we returned to the MHS's stated goal—to prepare health care leaders to succeed in joint, performance-based environments—and its desire to adopt a new paradigm for changing the way "we think and act," in particular to move to jointly staffed facilities, performance-based management, and total force and team development. We then looked for recommendations that would help transform leader development to meet the MHS's strategic goals.

Organizational Leader Expectations

- Reexamine the JMESP competency model to ensure that it meets the MHS's strategic goals, and infuse the competencies throughout the leader development process.
- Emphasize the importance of soft skills along with the hard skills in selection and evaluation.

How to Select

- Consider using performance-based interviews to recruit and evaluate officers for executive-level positions.
- Improve diversity among those selected for leader development opportunities.
- Implement a policy of "best in show" rather than "best in breed." In doing so, examine the health corps structure to ensure that all corps have equitable access to leadership opportunities.

How to Develop

- Reexamine the overall approach to leader development to determine whether it is feasible to provide shorter-term projects or stretch assignments to high-potentials.

- Provide physicians with leader development opportunities along with business and management skills earlier in their careers.
- Encourage the use of 360-degree feedback, and make it an integrated part of leader development.
- Examine ways of providing and validating shorter-term and more tailored joint training and education opportunities for health professions officers.
- Recognize the importance of mentoring in evaluations, and consider providing formal training in mentoring and coaching.
- Evaluate leader development programs for currency and relevancy.

How to Incentivize

- Consider a separate evaluation process or form for health professions officers that integrates the competencies that the military considers important. At the same time, consider ways to reduce subjectivity and inflation in evaluations.
- Examine ways of implementing three-year assignments for health professions officers.

We recognize that many of these approaches will require structural changes and may be difficult to implement. In addition, some may require difficult trade-offs. For example, selecting physicians for early leader development opportunities requires selecting fewer of them and necessarily narrowing the pipeline. This may result in overlooking some officers who have the potential to be effective leaders but who may not have the opportunity to distinguish themselves early in their careers. Going to three-year assignments has the same potential downside. Emphasizing joint education and training may mean reducing emphasis on other necessary management or leadership skills and training. Nonetheless, the recommendations here provide a useful starting point for discussion of how best to align leader development of health professions officers with the MHS's vision for transformation.

Acknowledgments

This study was supported and overseen by the flag officer steering committee and the executive integrated process team overseeing establishment of the joint medical education and training campus at Fort Sam Houston, Texas, as part of the transformation of the MHS mandated by the Quadrennial Defense Review. Both the steering committee and the executive integrated process team include senior representatives from each service, the Joint Staff, and U.S. Joint Forces Command. We are grateful to them for their guidance and support of the study.

We owe a debt of gratitude to our many respondents, without whose generous assistance the study could not have been completed. We are grateful to the military officers who participated in interviews and provided thoughtful comments and advice on how best to develop leaders for MHS positions. We are equally grateful to the many civilian and VHA senior leaders who took time out of their busy schedules to talk with us about their organizations' approaches to leader development and to share information about best practices.

Several current and former RAND colleagues contributed to the study. In particular, we thank our reviewers, Chaitra Hardison and Peter Schirmer. They not only provided critical and insightful reviews of the report but also gave us excellent suggestions for improving the clarity, flow, and readability of this monograph. We thank former RAND colleagues Marisa Adelson, Anant Patel, and Amber Price for their invaluable research assistance and enthusiasm. Robert Cox and then-LTC Jean Jones, a RAND Arroyo Center Army research fellow, contributed to an early phase of the study. Susan Hosek and Terri Tanielian provided useful comments as the study progressed and reviewed earlier drafts of this monograph. We are also grateful to Lauren Skrabala, our editor, for her impeccable editing, patience, and good humor.

Abbreviations

ACHE	American College of Healthcare Executives
ACPE	American College of Physician Executives
AFMS	U.S. Air Force Medical Service
AMEDD	U.S. Army Medical Department
AONE	American Organization of Nurse Executives
BSC	U.S. Air Force Biomedical Sciences Corps
BUMED	U.S. Navy Bureau of Medicine and Surgery
CEO	chief executive officer
CFO	chief financial officer
CNO	chief nursing officer
CO	commanding officer
COO	chief operating officer
DC	Dental Corps
DCA	deputy commander for administration
DLO	designated learning officer
DoD	U.S. Department of Defense
ECFCDP	Executive Career Field Candidate Development Program
FY	fiscal year
GS	General Schedule
HCA	Hospital Corporation of America

HLA	Healthcare Leadership Alliance
HPDM	High Performance Development Model
HR	human resource
ILE	intermediate-level education
JDAL	Joint Duty Assignment List
JMESI	Joint Medical Executive Skills Institute
JMESP	Joint Medical Executive Skills Program
JPME	joint professional military education
LEAD	Leadership, Effectiveness, Accountability, Development
LENS	Leadership Excellence Networks
MC	Medical Corps
MEDCOM	U.S. Army Medical Command
MHS	Military Health System
MSC	Medical Service Corps
MTF	medical treatment facility
NC	Nurse Corps
NCHL	National Center for Healthcare Leadership
NCOD	National Center for Organizational Development
NDRI	RAND National Defense Research Institute
NLB	National Leadership Board
OER	officer evaluation report
PBI	performance-based interviewing
PHS	U.S. Public Health Service
PME	professional military education
QDR	Quadrennial Defense Review
ROTC	Reserve Officers' Training Corps
SOARS	Systematic Ongoing Assessment and Review Strategy

SP	U.S. Army Medical Specialist Corps
VA	U.S. Department of Veterans Affairs
VC	U.S. Army Veterinary Corps
VHA	Veterans Health Administration
VHACO	Veterans Health Administration Central Office
VISN	Veterans Integrated Service Network
XO	executive officer

CHAPTER ONE

Introduction

The Military Health System (MHS), operated by the U.S. Department of Defense (DoD), is a $37-billion-a-year enterprise whose mission is "to enhance the Department of Defense and our Nation's security by providing health support for the full range of military operations and sustaining the health of all those entrusted to our care" (MHS, 2007a, p. 3). The full range of operations includes not only the more traditional military operations but also expanded DoD roles in security, stability, transition, and reconstruction operations,[1] as well as the provision of a range of military support to civil authorities.

The mission of the MHS has three components:

1. "Provide a medically ready and protected force and medical protection for communities" by continuously monitoring health status, identifying medical threats, and finding ways to provide protection and improve the health of individuals, communities, and the nation.
2. "Create a deployable medical capability that can go anywhere, anytime with flexibility, interoperability, and agility," to assist in a wide range of military and civil support operations (including homeland defense).
3. "Manage and deliver a superb health benefit" to members of the armed forces, their dependents, and others entitled to DoD medical care through an integrated health delivery system that "encompasses military treatment facilities,[2] private sector care, and other federal health facilities" (MHS, 2007a, p. 14).

Over the past few years, there has been increasing recognition that the MHS has to transform itself and the way it does business. This recognition has been driven by the

---

[1] DoD Directive 3000.5 (2005, para. 4.1) clearly states,

> Stability operations are a core U.S. military mission that the Department of Defense shall be prepared to conduct and support. They shall be given priority comparable to combat operations and be explicitly addressed and integrated across all DoD activities including doctrine, organizations, training, education, exercises, materiel, leadership, personnel, facilities, and planning.

[2] *Medical treatment facility* (MTF) refers to any medical care site, such as a clinic, hospital, or medical center.

rapid escalation in the costs of health care, a changing environment with an increased emphasis on performance management, the unprecedented challenges faced by the U.S. military at home and abroad that require it to assume new roles and responsibilities, and the need to transform the medical force so that future medical support is fully aligned with joint force concepts. For example, the 2006 Quadrennial Defense Review (QDR) and, more specifically, the MHS QDR Roadmap for Medical Transformation (MHS, 2006) highlighted the importance of preparing health care leaders to succeed in joint, performance-based environments (see DoD, 2006). The 2008 MHS Strategic Plan pointed to the need to change the culture of the MHS in profound ways and to adopt a new paradigm for doing business:

> To achieve a true transformation and the breakthrough performance we desire, we must transform our culture in profound ways. Our culture is defined by the assumptions and mental models we use to understand the world and guide our behaviors. (MHS, 2008)

We reproduce the detailed MHS plan for transformation in Table 1.1.

Table 1.1
MHS Plan for Transformation

Old Paradigm	New Paradigm
Why should we . . . ?	Why couldn't we . . . ?
Two competing missions, health care delivery and force health protection	One mission, three interdependent themes
Service-specific infrastructure	Jointly staffed facilities
Budget and rules based	Performance-based management
End year with no money left	End year with savings and meet performance goals
Beneficiary satisfaction surveys	Customer relationship building
Provider centered	Patient control and accountability
Direct care system of MTFs and network of civilian providers	Integrated health delivery team with shared accountability
Proprietary information	Data sharing
Fixed-fee contracts	Performance-based contracting
Active duty, reserve, guard, civilians, and contractors managed separately	Total force and team development

SOURCE: MHS, 2008, p. 6.

Purpose of This Study

This study was part of a larger project conducted by the RAND National Defense Research Institute to assist the MHS in establishing a joint medical education and training campus at Fort Sam Houston, Texas, pursuant to the recommendations of the Base Realignment and Closure Commission to provide training in enlisted medical specialties in the Army, Navy, and Air Force. The establishment of the campus is being overseen by an executive integrated process team under the guidance of a tri-service flag officer steering committee. As part of this project, RAND was asked to examine the ways in which senior leaders in the medical field are prepared and supported in the civilian and military sectors, to review the competencies necessary to be a leader in the current performance-based and joint environment, and to recommend ways to enhance and transform military health care leader training. At the outset, we should note that we use the term *leader* to identify an individual who is likely to be in a command or executive position in an organization; on the military side, this refers to senior officers at the O-6 level and above.

The study included a review of the literature on leader development, structured interviews with civilian and military health care leaders and managers, and a case study of how one government agency—the Veterans Health Administration (VHA)—approaches executive leader development. The VHA was selected because of both its similarity to and close ties with the military services and its systematic approach to leader development. The study results offer a rich and detailed portrait of how three sectors—military, civilian, and government—develop health care leaders.

This monograph focuses on the following topics:

- the ways in which leader competencies are outlined and used in selected civilian, government, and military health organizations
- the strengths and weaknesses in the current system's ability to produce successful leaders for today's performance-based and joint environments
- lessons learned from civilian and other government agencies with respect to best practices for developing leaders.

An additional task of the larger project was to examine the feasibility of qualifying health professions officers[3] as "joint" officers. As noted earlier, there is increasing recognition that the roles that the MHS is being asked to play, especially with

---

[3] Following DoD Directive 6000.12 (1996), we use the term *health professions officers* when referring to officers who are "serving in the Medical Corps, the Dental Corps, the Veterinary Corps, the Nurse Corps, the Medical Service Corps, the Army Medical Specialist Corps, the Biomedical Sciences Corps, officers whom the Secretaries of the Military Departments have designated as 'qualified in specified healthcare functions,' and those members in DoD programs leading to commissioning in, assignment to, or designation for service in any of those Corps" (Enclosure 2). When referring more generally to leaders in the civilian and military sectors and in the VHA, we use the term *health care leaders*.

respect to national emergencies (such as pandemic influenza) and reconstruction operations, require working strategically with other nations, other militaries, and other
agencies—in other words, understanding and functioning in joint environments,
where *joint* includes multiservice, interagency, intergovernmental, and multinational
arrangements. However, there are several barriers to providing health professions officers with joint education and experience, which are more fully discussed in an earlier
RAND publication (Kirby and Thie, 2009). Here, we provide service respondents'
views regarding the value of joint education, experience, and skills for military health
professions officers.

Research Questions

The study was designed to address the following research questions:

1. What are the competencies required of leaders in the health care field?
2. What is the current career path for officers in health care professions in the
   three services? How does this path differ across the various corps and services?
   How are current leaders supported in terms of provision of needed professional
   development and career counseling or mentoring?
3. What are officers' perceptions about how well the current system works in preparing health care leaders to succeed in performance-based and joint environments? What are the gaps and perceived problems in the current system's ability
   to produce successful leaders for today's world?
4. What lessons can be learned from civilian health care organizations in terms of
   leader development?
5. What lessons can be learned from the case study of the VHA?

We developed a conceptual framework to guide our data collection and analysis.
An important aspect of the task included examining and summarizing the competencies that military, civilian, and VHA organizations expect of leaders in the health care
field—our first research question. To address the second and third research questions,
we interviewed military health care leaders in the three services. To address questions
four and five, we undertook a series of interviews with senior leaders in civilian health
care organizations and associations and in the VHA. Our data and methods are more
fully described in Chapter Two.

To set the context for the study, we first provide some background on the military
components of the MHS and a profile of the military health care officer workforce by
service, corps, and rank.

Overview of the Military Health System

The MHS encompasses five entities:[4] Health Affairs, TRICARE Management Activity, and the medical components of the Army, Navy,[5] and Air Force. The service medical components contribute to the MHS readiness mission by operating MTFs; recruiting, equipping, and training the medical force; and supporting operational readiness through force health protection. The Army, Navy, and Air Force individually staff the service-specific MTFs with active-duty, reserve, and federal civilian medical workforces. In addition to recruitment and retention, the services provide education, leadership development, and other training programs to support MHS needs (MHS, 2007b, p. 6).

Military health care in the services is provided by their respective medical divisions, the U.S. Army Medical Department (AMEDD), the U.S. Navy Bureau of Medicine and Surgery (BUMED), and the U.S. Air Force Medical Service (AFMS). Unlike the AFMS, "AMEDD and BUMED maintain command of the Medical Force, deploy mission support in theater, and provide beneficiary medical care" (MHS, 2007b, p. 6). However, in the Air Force, similar medical responsibilities are under the command of the line.

U.S. Army Medical Department

AMEDD's mission is to promote, sustain, and enhance soldier health; train, develop, and equip a medical force that supports full-spectrum operations; and deliver leading-edge health services to warriors and military families to optimize outcomes (AMEDD, 2010). AMEDD administers eight medical centers, 26 medical departments, and numerous clinics;[6] cares for more than 5 million active-duty personnel, retirees, and family members; and had a budget of $9.7 billion in 2006.

The Army Surgeon General heads both AMEDD and the U.S. Army Medical Command (MEDCOM). As the head of AMEDD, the Surgeon General advises the Secretary of the Army on medical affairs; as the head of MEDCOM, the Surgeon General commands hospitals and other AMEDD commands and agencies.

---

[4] This section draws heavily on the *MHS Human Capital Strategic Plan, 2008–2013* (MHS, 2007b, pp. 6–8).

[5] The Navy is responsible for medical care in both the Navy and the Marine Corps.

[6] Clinics are outpatient facilities offering primary care or simple specialty care, such as routine exams, tests, and treatments. A clinic may be a stand-alone site or part of a major health facility (a family-practice clinic, pediatric clinic, etc., within a hospital). Medical centers offer tertiary care (sophisticated diagnosis and treatment), as well as primary and secondary care; they provide hospital care and other services (e.g., preventive medicine, blood bank). An Army Medical Department Activity is a medical command-and-control headquarters at a given post and typically includes one community hospital or clinic plus nonhospital elements (e.g., preventive medicine, blood bank) (AMEDD, 2008).

Within the Army, medical human capital management functions are centralized and are the responsibility of three subcomponents of AMEDD:

the Human Resources Directorate, which manages the people within the Army; the AMEDD Proponency Office, which manages billets, recruiting, and retention; and the Program Analysis & Evaluation within the office of the Secretary General, which plans for resource integration and transition, program analysis, and evaluation capabilities for effective resource management of enterprise-wide programs. (MHS, 2007b, p. 6)

U.S. Navy Bureau of Medicine and Surgery

BUMED's mission is "to be ready to care for those in need, anytime, anywhere." BUMED personnel provide mission support on ships, in the air, and on the battlefield. BUMED oversees 22 hospitals, three naval medical commands, six clinics, and 11 dental centers; provides care to 2.6 million beneficiaries; and had a budget of $5.7 billion in 2006.

Like the Army Surgeon General, the Navy Surgeon General serves as both the director of naval medicine and head of BUMED, advising the Chief of Naval Operations on naval health service programs and overseeing all systems providing health services to beneficiaries during peacetime and wartime.

As in the Army,

[h]uman capital management functions within Navy Medicine are centralized and carried out by the Human Resources Department of BUMED, which develops and directs Navy Medicine manpower plans and personnel policies. The department is responsible for developing staff standards, analyzing and evaluating Total Medical Force planning and programming for acquisition and alignment, developing proposals to achieve required Total Medical Force structure, coordinating Navy Medicine's personnel actions in relation to the DoD, and acting as the functional sponsor for manpower and personnel information systems. (MHS, 2007b, p. 7)

U.S. Air Force Medical Service

The AFMS's mission is to provide "seamless health service support to the [Air Force] and combatant commanders. The AFMS assists in sustaining the performance, health and fitness of every Airman" (Air Force Surgeon General, undated). The AFMS has 74 MTFs, 11 hospitals, three medical centers, and two medical wings. It provides care to more than 2.6 million beneficiaries and had a budget of $6.9 billion in 2006.

The AFMS directly supports Air Force operations and theater aeromedical evacuation of joint and combined forces. In addition, the Air Force Surgeon General is responsible for developing and implementing medical programs and policies that provide for the health care of military personnel and their family members.

Unlike the Army and Navy,

Air Force human capital functions are unique because they are decentralized and managed within the commands and MTFs. However, human capital strategy and direction on personnel requirements come from AF/A1, the personnel and manpower portion of the entire Air Force. When individuals join the AFMS they are assigned to specific MTFs by the Air Force Personnel Center. MTFs provide the decentralized human capital functions and administer human capital programs at a local level. (MHS, 2007b, p. 8)

Profile of Health Professions Officers in the Military Health System

To set the context for the next several chapters, we provide a profile of health professions officers serving in the AMEDD, BUMED, and AFMS in terms of specialty and grade. All three services have a Medical Corps (MC), Dental Corps (DC), Nurse Corps (NC), and Medical Service Corps (MSC). However, the definition of MSC specialties differs across the three services. For example, the Army MSC encompasses specialists in behavioral sciences, laboratory sciences, optometry, pharmacy, podiatry, and preventive medicine sciences, as well as health care administrators, while the Navy MSC includes not only these specialties but also occupational therapists, physical therapists, dieticians, and physician assistants. In the Army, these latter specialties are grouped under the Army Medical Specialist Corps (SP). The Air Force limits its MSC officers to those specializing in health care administration and finance. All other specialties listed above are grouped under the Air Force Biomedical Sciences Corps (BSC). The other major difference is that the Army has a small Veterinary Corps (VC) comprising fewer than 500 officers, which is involved in animal medicine, public health, food inspection, and research and development.

Table 1.2 shows the distribution of officers by corps and service from fiscal year (FY) 2004 through FY 2008. For each year, we show the absolute (number of officers) and relative (percentage of total) size of the corps by service. The last column shows the percentage change in the size of the corps from FY 2004 to FY 2008. The total health professions officer end strength in the three services declined 4 percent over the five-year period, from 37,001 in September 2004 to 35,475 in September 2008 (not shown). This decline was primarily due to declines in Navy and Air Force end strength (9 percent and 12 percent, respectively, over this period). In contrast, the Army experienced a 6-percent gain in health care officer end strength. In FY 2008, the Army accounted for 42 percent of all health professions officers, the Navy for 28 percent, and the Air Force for 31 percent.

Table 1.2
Five-Year Summary of Active-Duty Health Professions Officer End Strength, by Service, Corps, and Fiscal Year

Corps	FY 2004		FY 2005		FY 2006		FY 2007		FY 2008		% Change, FY 2004– FY 2008
	N	%	N	%	N	%	N	%	N	%	
Army											
Medical	4,230	30.5	4,243	30.7	4,253	30.3	4,274	29.8	4,309	29.2	1.9
Dental	957	6.9	944	6.8	932	6.6	933	6.5	928	6.3	–3.0
Nurse	3,157	22.7	3,089	22.3	3,134	22.3	3,241	22.6	3,367	22.8	6.7
Medical Service	4,025	29.0	4,070	29.4	4,137	29.5	4,312	30.0	4,423	29.9	9.9
Medical Specialist	1,095	7.9	1,062	7.7	1,130	8.1	1,175	8.2	1,299	8.8	18.6
Veterinary	424	3.1	433	3.1	443	3.2	430	3.0	445	3.0	5.0
Total	13,888	100.0	13,841	100.0	14,029	100.0	14,365	100.0	14,771	100.0	6.4
Navy											
Medical	3,952	36.5	3,845	37.0	3,811	37.9	3,730	37.9	3,762	38.2	–4.8
Dental	1,205	11.1	1,130	10.9	1,058	10.5	1,008	10.3	1,001	10.2	–16.9
Nurse	3,038	28.1	2,934	28.2	2,829	28.1	2,803	28.5	2,795	28.4	–8.0
Medical Service	2,627	24.3	2,490	23.9	2,363	23.5	2,293	23.3	2,278	23.2	–13.3
Total	10,822	100.0	10,399	100.0	10,061	100.0	9,834	100.0	9,836	100.0	–9.1
Air Force											
Medical	3,602	29.3	3,544	30.0	3,452	31.0	3,429	31.7	3,459	31.8	–4.0
Dental	1,010	8.2	961	8.1	927	8.3	901	8.3	922	8.5	–8.7
Nurse	3,733	30.4	3,529	29.9	3,429	30.8	3,289	30.4	3,276	30.1	–12.2
Medical Service	1,392	11.3	1,392	11.8	1,116	10.0	1,071	9.9	1,029	9.5	–26.1
Biomedical Sciences	2,554	20.8	2,380	20.2	2,222	19.9	2,133	19.7	2,182	20.1	–14.6
Total	12,291	100.0	11,806	100.0	11,146	100.0	10,823	100.0	10,868	100.0	–11.6

NOTE: N = number of officers. Percentages may not add to 100 due to rounding.

Looking now at the relative distribution of officer end strength by corps as of September 2008 (Table 1.2), we find the following:

- In the Army, the MC and MSC both accounted for 29–30 percent of all health professions officers in FY 2008, followed by the NC (23 percent). About 9 percent of health professions officers were in the SP, and about 6 percent in the DC. The SP experienced a relatively large increase in end strength over time (19 percent), while the gains experienced by the MSC and NC were somewhat smaller (10 percent and 7 percent, respectively). In contrast, the MC increased by 2 percent, while the DC experienced a small decline (3 percent). The VC—which is relatively small, as noted earlier—increased by 5 percent over this period and accounted for 3 percent of health professions officers in FY 2008.
- In the Navy, about 38 percent of all health professions officers were in the MC, followed by 28 percent in the NC and 23 percent in the MSC in FY 2008. The DC accounted for 10 percent of all health professions officers. All the corps experienced declines in end strength, ranging from 17 percent in the DC to 5 percent in the MC. The MSC and NC declined by 13 percent and 8 percent, respectively.
- The two largest corps in the Air Force were the MC and NC, each accounting for 30–32 percent of health professions officers in FY 2008. About 20 percent of health professions officers were in the BSC, and another 10 percent were in the MSC. As with the Navy, all the corps suffered declines in end strength, and the MSC was the hardest hit, experiencing a decline of 26 percent over the five-year period. The BSC and NC decreased by 12–15 percent, while the DC and MC had the smallest declines, 9 percent and 4 percent, respectively.

Table 1.3 presents the grade distribution of the health care officer force by service and corps as of the end of FY 2008. For each service and corps, we show the relative distribution of officers by grade. Thus, of 4,309 Army MC officers, 42 percent were junior officers in grades O-1 through O-3. Across the three services, the DC tended to be the most senior: Twenty-one percent of Air Force and 24 percent of Army and Navy DC officers were at the O-6 or flag officer level, followed by the MC (10–12 percent). Only 3–5 percent of nurses were at the O-6 level or higher, as were 5–8 percent of the MSC officers, 2 percent of the Army SP officers, and 4 percent of Air Force BSC officers. About 8 percent of the VC were O-6s or higher. Flag officers are drawn primarily from the MC. For example, of the 15 Army flag officers, 11 were in the MC, while the DC, NC, MSC, and VC had one each. Of the 16 Navy flag officers, 12 were in the MC, while the DC and MSC had one each and the NC had two. Of the 13 Air Force flag officers, nine were in the MC, and there was one in each of remaining corps (one each in the DC, NC, MSC, and BSC).

Table 1.3
Active-Duty Health Professions Officer End Strength, by Service, Corps, and Officer Grade, September 2008

Corps	Percentage of Total in Corps					Total Health Professions Officers
	O-1 to O-3	O-4	O-5	O-6	O-7 to O-9	
Army						
Medical	41.8	30.0	16.3	11.7	0.3	4,309
Dental	47.1	15.1	14.1	23.6	0.1	928
Nurse	64.5	20.0	11.7	3.9	0.0[a]	3,367
Medical Service	61.9	20.6	12.4	5.1	0.0[a]	4,423
Medical Specialist	73.5	18.6	5.8	2.1	0.0	1,299
Veterinary	40.2	33.5	18.2	7.9	0.2	445
Total (number)	8,280	3,408	1,931	1,137	15[a]	14,771
Navy						
Medical	38.1	31.6	19.3	10.7	0.3	3,762
Dental	36.2	18.9	20.6	24.3	0.1	1,001
Nurse	58.7	23.1	13.4	4.7	0.1	2,795
Medical Service	54.7	24.1	14.2	7.0	0.0[a]	2,278
Total (number)	4,683	2,570	1,632	935	16[a]	9,836
Air Force						
Medical	40.2	31.5	18.8	9.2	0.3	3,459
Dental	41.3	16.8	20.5	21.3	0.1	922
Nurse	61.7	25.8	9.7	2.8	0.0[a]	3,276
Medical Service	43.9	27.4	21.0	7.6	0.1	1,029
Biomedical Sciences	47.5	32.5	16.0	4.0	0.0[a]	2,182
Total (number)	5,281	3,081	1,722	771	13[a]	10,868

[a] Accounted for less than 0.05% of total health professions officers.

Organization of This Monograph

The next chapter presents the conceptual model that we used to structure our interviews and to organize our VHA case study. It also lays out the competencies required of military health professionals, addressing our first research question. It concludes with a discussion of our data sources and how we analyzed the data. Chapters Three and Four address the second and third research questions. Chapter Three describes how military health care leaders are developed: how they enter the service and how they are developed within a life-cycle model for each military service. That chapter provides some context for the material gathered in our interviews with military personnel. Chapter Four presents the results of our interviews with military health care professionals. Chapter Five focuses on the fourth research question, presenting the results of our interviews with civilian health care leaders and drawing lessons learned about leader development on the civilian side. Chapter Six discusses the VHA case study to address the fifth research question. In addition to presenting findings from interviews with a wide variety of VHA personnel, that chapter also outlines the VHA's evolution over the past decade and presents information from numerous documents with respect to how the VHA approaches leader development. Chapter Seven presents our conclusions and recommendations.

This monograph includes seven appendixes. Appendix A provides additional material on how we selected our sample of civilian health care organizations. Appendix B contains an overview of the joint professional military education (JPME) available to line officers and health professionals. Appendixes C, D, and E, respectively, contain additional material from the interviews we conducted with Army, Navy, and Air Force officers. Appendixes F and G provide additional information about educational opportunities and programs offers by civilian health care organizations and the VHA, respectively.

CHAPTER TWO

Conceptual Framework, Data, and Methods

We developed a conceptual framework to guide our data collection and analysis. This chapter describes that framework and explains its components and the sources that influenced our construction of the framework. We use the conceptual framework as a way of organizing the material drawn from our interviews with military health professionals from the three services and the civilian health care organizations in our sample and to characterize the VHA's approach to developing its executives. The second part of the chapter outlines the data we gathered and the methods we used to analyze them.

Conceptual Framework

Based on a review of the literature on leader development and competency frameworks, we developed a conceptual framework for modeling leader development of military health professions officers to guide our data collection and analysis.[1] Although the framework is couched in generic terms that apply to the civilian sector as well, our focus here is on how the military identifies and develops its senior leaders for MHS positions. This framework is presented in Figure 2.1.

One of the primary goals of the officer management system—the box labeled "outcome" in the figure—is to produce qualified senior leaders who can function in both joint and service-specific environments and who possess the competencies determined to be important for successful leadership. Our framework assumes that military health professions officers are functionally qualified and continue to develop their domain knowledge and skills through continuing education ("input"). Thus, our focus is on who is developed and where and how these officers receive the knowledge, experience, and acculturation necessary to qualify them for leadership in both service and joint environments. The conceptual framework does not consider those who are on a long-term clinical or academic track, and who may require different knowledge and experiences, but instead focuses on health professions officers likely to be in command positions.

---

[1]   Again, the term *leader* refers to an individual who is likely to be in a command or executive position in the organization.

Figure 2.1
Conceptual Framework for Leader Development

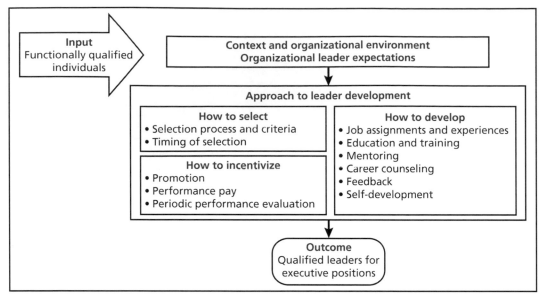

Context and Organizational Environment

An organization's approach to leader development plays out against the larger backdrop of the local, regional, national, and global context, which can shape what an organization expects from leaders and how it designs and implements development strategies. These contextual factors also enable or constrain an organization's ability to develop needed leaders. For example, increased competition from other sectors, the demands of wartime and frequent deployments, and changes in the way in which health care professionals are paid and rewarded could have important implications for an organization's ability to recruit, develop, and retain the caliber of individual it desires. In addition, the overall organizational environment—the structure, policies, and culture of the organization—directly influences how leaders are developed and supported and the leader development strategies that the organization adopts. As McAlearney (2006) points out, an organization's commitment to leader development, which is driven by the organizational environment, "influences the program design process, resulting in broader or narrower leadership development opportunities for individuals" (p. 976). Thus, if leader development is not seen as central to the organization or is not fully supported by the top leadership, leader development strategies may not be well integrated into the organization's goals and objectives and may be underfunded as well. If succession planning or "deepening the bench" is not seen as vital to the organization, the organization will develop insufficient numbers of leaders who are committed to and steeped in its values and ethos. In this way, the organizational context determines the range, centrality, stability, and coherence of the leader development strategies adopted by the organization.

Organizational Expectations for Leaders

The conceptual framework presented in Figure 2.1 also assumes that organizations have explicit and implicit expectations for their leaders that often guide development efforts.[2] Some organizations formalize these expectations into a set of competencies or competency models. In some cases, expectations may be reflected in evaluation and promotion criteria, compensation policies, job descriptions, or training curricula.

To determine the kinds of skills and experience that health care organizations generally believe that leaders need, we reviewed a number of civilian health care leadership competency frameworks (from the National Center for Healthcare Leadership [NCHL], the Healthcare Leadership Alliance [HLA], and the National Public Health Leadership Development Network)[3] and military health care leadership competencies—in particular, the 39 competencies outlined by the Joint Medical Executive Skills Program (JMESP)—deemed important for military medical executives across the services.[4] As described on the website of the JMESI, which oversees the JMESP, "The 39 competencies are the primary knowledge, skills, abilities, [and] attitudes determined necessary for successful command of a medical treatment facility or other executive medicine position within the MHS, such as a lead agent, or executive officer" (JMESI, undated). The JMESP competencies overlap to a considerable extent with those established by the leading civilian professional organizations.

Underlying traits not explicitly listed in the following competency models but that some literature has noted as important are personal integrity, moral character, and commitment to organizational values. Often, these characteristics seem to be implicit in discussions of traits and skills needed for health care leaders, which tend to focus largely on those traits and skills that can be learned or enhanced (although competencies like creativity, flexibility, and adaptability are arguably more inherent than learned).

NCHL Health Leadership Competency Model (Version 2.0). The NCHL Health Leadership Competency Model (Version 2.0) builds on research conducted for the earlier model developed in 2003 as well as behavioral observation (including behavioral event interviews and one-on-one interviews) and modeling methods (such as database benchmarking). The model defines competency as "those behavioral and techni-

---

[2] See Brannman et al. (2007) for an excellent review of leader competency frameworks, an annotated bibliography of the literature on leader development, and a description of selected service courses aimed at providing military leaders with the needed executive skills.

[3] Additional competency models have also been developed for specific jobs within the health professions, including clinical management, nursing, and public health (see Calhoun et al., 2008).

[4] The Joint Medical Executive Skills Institute (JMESI) was established in 1998 as an executive agency to oversee the services' medical executive education programs and to be a proponent for JMESP. JMESI is under the authority of the Army Surgeon General (see JMESI, undated).

cal characteristics that discriminate outstanding leadership performance from typical performance across the health professions" (Calhoun et al., 2008, p. 337). It includes 26 competencies under the following three domains:

- The *transformation* domain includes achievement orientation, analytical thinking, community orientation, financial skills, information seeking, innovative thinking, and strategic orientation.
- The *execution* domain includes accountability, change leadership, collaboration, communication skills, impact and influence, information technology management, initiative, organizational awareness, performance measurement, process management and organizational design, and project management.
- The *people* domain includes human resource (HR) management, interpersonal understanding, professionalism, relationship building, self-confidence, self-development, talent development, and team leadership (Brannman et al., 2007; Calhoun et al., 2008).

Of the 26 competencies, eight are technical: financial skills, strategic orientation, communication skills, information technology management, performance measurement, process management and organizational design, project management, and HR management (Brannman et al., 2007; Calhoun et al., 2008).

Competencies are scaled to describe the different levels of performance as roles and responsibilities increase in scope, complexity, and sophistication (Calhoun et al., 2008). Each competency is defined with three to six levels of specified behaviors. For example, the accountability competency encompasses five levels. Outstanding early-career individuals perform at a level 3, whereas outstanding midcareer and advanced-career individuals perform at level 4 and level 5, respectively (Calhoun et al., 2008). This competency model provides a conceptual basis to assess individual needs for improvement, to design education and training opportunities, and to facilitate a systems-based approach of organizational design (Baker, 2003; Brannman et al., 2007; Calhoun et al., 2008).

HLA Competency Directory. The American College of Healthcare Executives (ACHE), in conjunction with other members of the HLA,[5] created the HLA Competency Directory, a searchable reference tool that allows users to filter and sort information by domain, competency, skill area, management specialty, and keywords (Baker, 2003; Brannman et al., 2007; HLA, 2005). Based on job analyses and research to validate the components, the directory includes 300 skill-oriented competencies iden-

---

[5]   The HLA members are the ACHE, American College of Physician Executives (ACPE), American Organization of Nurse Executives (AONE), Healthcare Financial Management Association, Healthcare Information Management Systems Society, Medical Group Management Association, and American College of Medical Practice Executives (the certifying body of the Medical Group Management Association). However, the ACPE did not participate in the HLA Competency Directory effort. See HLA (undated) for more information.

tified as important across diverse professional roles in the health care management field (Brannman et al., 2007; HLA, 2005). Competencies are categorized into five domains:

- The *communication and relationship management* competency domain refers to the skills and capabilities needed to communicate clearly and concisely with internal and external customers, to establish and maintain relationships, and to facilitate constructive interactions with others.
- The *leadership* domain is defined by the ability to inspire individual and organizational excellence, to create a shared vision, and to successfully manage change to achieve organizational strategic goals.
- *Professionalism* refers to the skills and capabilities of aligning personal and organizational conduct with ethical and professional standards.
- *Knowledge of the health care environment* is the demonstration of understanding of the health care system and the environment in which health care organizations and professionals function.
- The *business knowledge and skills* domain includes financial management, HR, organizational dynamics and governance, strategic planning and marketing, information management, risk management, and quality improvement (Brannman et al., 2007; HLA, 2005).

The HLA Competency Directory can be used for job descriptions, self-assessment, development and improvement of certification programs, curriculum design for health care leadership training and education, and organizational analysis and strategic planning (Brannman et al., 2007; HLA, 2005).

Military Health Care Leader Competencies. Pursuant to a 1992 congressional mandate that MTF commanders must possess certain executive competencies before assuming command positions, DoD and the services established a joint medical executive skills development program (now the JMESP) to prepare MHS officers for executive duties. The program encompassed 40 (reduced to 39 in 2008) executive competencies that military health care officers must possess (JMESI, 2008). These 39 competencies are organized into seven domains: military medical, leadership and organizational management, health law and policy, health resource allocation, ethics in the health care environment, individual and organizational behavior, and performance measurement and improvement. Because these 39 competencies are central to the development of military health care leaders, we describe them, by domain, in Table 2.1.

The JMESP competencies have considerable overlap with civilian competencies, with the obvious exception of the competencies that characterize the military medical domain specifically, those that are unique to the military, and some that are not relevant to the military at all (for example, negotiating salary compensation for physicians).

Table 2.1
Joint Medical Executive Skills, 2008

Domain	Competencies
Military medical	*Medical doctrine* refers to the fundamental principles that are used to guide medical forces' actions in support of military objectives.
	Military mission entails the understanding, provision, and evaluation of health service support for military operational requirements.
	Joint operations require participation in individual, collective, and unit medical readiness training that includes joint and combined exercises or deployment.
	Total force management refers to doctrine and procedures for management of all military medical components.
	Medical readiness training includes courses, hands-on training programs, and exercises designed to ensure proper functioning of health care personnel and units.
	Disaster and contingency planning refers to the preparation for delivery of medical services in unanticipated events involving military forces and includes readiness planning, organization, management, logistics, personnel, and patient care.
Leadership and organizational management	*Strategic planning* refers to the capabilities of managing the iterative organizational process for assessing a situation, establishing strategic goals, and implementing strategic plans in support of mission requirements.
	Organizational design refers to the capabilities of evaluating and optimizing the configuration of an organization's design elements, such as personnel, organizational structure, tasks, technology, processes, mission, and values.
	Decisionmaking is the skill of selecting appropriate courses of action from alternatives.
	Change and innovation refers to the abilities to recognize the need for innovation, develop proper strategies for change, and implement the strategies successfully.
	Leadership is the art and science of motivating people to act toward accomplishing a mission.
Health law and policy	*Public law* includes regulations in areas such as public health, patient consent and rights, and environmental standards.
	Medical liability refers to tort and criminal offenses that may incur risk to health care providers.
	Medical staff by-laws concern the conduct and privileges of the medical staff.
	Regulations include all federal, state, and local policies that affect a health care organization's operation.
	External accreditation is an evaluation process performed by an accrediting organization to review the health care delivery practices of a medical facility.
Health resource allocation	*Financial management* refers to the use of analytical techniques to ensure adequate resources to meet the health care organization's mission.
	HR management includes staffing, management, and retention of personnel.
	Labor-management relations refers to the interactions between the organization's management and civilian staff, such as collective bargaining, implementation of fair labor practices, and grievance management.
	Materiel management refers to medical logistics, i.e., the management of supplies and equipment.
	Facilities management is the maintenance and upkeep of real property, such as a building, structure, or utility system.
	Information management and technology refers to the principles and techniques for the use of information and technology in support of readiness and business processes.

Table 2.1—Continued

Domain	Competencies
Ethics in the health care environment	*Ethical foundations* includes an understanding of the processes, structures, and social constructs by which rightness or wrongness of actions is assessed and the process of resolving ethical dilemmas.
	Personal and professional ethics includes having a personal and professional code of ethics and identifying and addressing ethical conflicts between personal values and professional ethical standards.
	Bioethics represents the application of normative ethics to the life sciences and includes clinical ethics and, more broadly, the general application of ethics through policy.
	Organizational ethics describes the structures and processes by which an organization ensures conduct appropriate to its mission and vision.
Individual and organizational behavior	*Individual behavior* refers to the influence of the leader's behavior and personality on the organization.
	Group dynamics is the use of interactions among organization members to facilitate effective group behavior.
	Conflict management involves the identification and use of techniques to effectively manage conflicts.
	Communication refers to the ability to choose appropriate communication styles and media, to convey messages clearly and effectively, and to solicit and incorporate feedback.
	Public speaking refers to the verbal and organizing skills needed to effectively communicate to a wide range of audiences.
	Strategic communication involves the development and delivery of an effective and consistent message and encompasses media, public relations, and risk communication.
Performance measurement and improvement	*Epidemiological methods* include medical surveillance, interventions, and risk communication.
	Clinical investigation entails initiation, performance, completion, publication, and use of research.
	Integrated health care delivery systems provide health care options using partnerships with other DoD, U.S. Department of Veterans Affairs (VA), managed care support, and U.S. Public Health Service (PHS) organizations and all available health care delivery assets.
	Quality management refers to the procedures emphasizing involvement, empowerment, and continuous performance improvement.
	Quantitative and qualitative analysis is the use of analytical tools and methods for decisionmaking.
	Outcome measurements allow the health care leaders to make fact-based decisions.
	Patient safety involves all activities aimed at minimizing the risk of medical error.

SOURCE: JMESI, 2008.

Categorization of Organizational Leader Expectations. The leader skills and competencies identified by organizations define the "outcome" desired by organizations. (We distinguish between what is produced by the leader development system and what is desired by the organization, which are not necessarily the same.) These organizational expectations for leaders can be usefully categorized into leadership, management, and enterprise domains, regardless of sector or profession (Robbert, 2005). Organizations look for both competencies and experience (demonstrated use of these competencies). As Robbert (2005) points out, leadership skills "are honed through observation and practice—actual experience in seeking to shape the behaviors of organizations and the individuals within them, or in observing the efforts of others" (p. 262); management skills can be taught but atrophy unless practiced; and a "thorough understanding of the internal and external environments of an organization is typically gained through experience and mentoring" where the experience "might include serving in a variety of field and headquarters levels of the organization, as well as in the important operating environments of the organization" (p. 261).

First, *management knowledge and experience* includes the skills and abilities to manage financial, human, and information resources to ensure successful fulfillment of organizational goals. Identified common competencies that fall into this category include HR management (such as recruitment, staffing, mentoring and coaching, training, and evaluation and assessment), financial resource management (such as budgeting, asset management, and monitoring of the use of financial resources), information management and technology, and interpersonal and communication skills (with internal and external customers). Second, *leadership knowledge and experience* provides strategic and visionary guidance to help the organization meet future challenges. Competencies that fall into this category include visionary leadership (i.e., envisioning a future state and influencing movement toward it), change leadership (i.e., continuously seeking innovative approaches and welcoming changes as opportunities for improvement), and strategic thinking and planning. Finally, *enterprise knowledge and experience* includes competencies that demonstrate the sound understanding of the profession and the organization, such as organizational awareness, an understanding of the larger context in which the organization operates, and the global environment. Enterprise knowledge and experience is increasingly seen as important for military leaders as military operations become more joint and integrated (interservice, interagency, intergovernmental, and multinational). The *Capstone Concept for Joint Operations*, version 2.0 (DoD, 2005), which describes how the military will operate in the future as a joint force and provides a format for leader development, states that joint force leaders should be "knowledgeable, empowered, innovative, and decisive leaders, capable of leading the networked joint force to success in fluid and perhaps chaotic operating environments, with more comprehensive knowledge of interagency and foreign cultures and capabilities" (p. 24).

We can map the JMESP domains into these three categories, although, arguably, they often span more than one dimension. For example, health law and policy, health resource allocation, individual and organizational behavior, and performance measurement and improvement could be grouped under management knowledge; leadership and organizational management and ethics in the health care environment seem to equate to leadership knowledge; and the military medical domain falls under enterprise knowledge.

Approach to Leader Development

An organization's approach to leader development has three facets: whom to select for leader development and how; strategies for leader development; and how to incentivize the high-potentials whom the organization wishes to develop and retain. In terms of whom to select, the organization could choose to develop all midlevel managers or target selected groups identified as high-potentials. Selection could also be more happenstance, with higher-level education and training being offered to those who were available at the time, rather than to the best-qualified candidates. The selection process also encompasses strategies adopted by the organization for identifying potential leaders. These include formal means, such as requiring individuals to submit written applications of qualifications and establishing criteria for ranking the applications, interviews, and written letters of recommendations, or informal means, such as word of mouth from supervisors or peers.

Strategies for developing leaders include job assignments and experiences, education and training,[6] mentoring, career counseling, feedback, and self-development. Organizations differ in terms of how much emphasis they place on particular strategies and how systematically and purposefully they use these approaches to develop leaders. A review of industry best practices conducted by Day and Halpin (2001) for the U.S. Army identified a number of best practices in leader development, including

> formal development programs (which often include a number of other specific practices), 360-degree feedback (or multi-source ratings of performance), executive coaching (focused one-on-one learning), job assignments (to challenge or stretch an individual's leadership capabilities), mentoring (longer-term developmental relationships), networks (connecting to others across the organization's internal boundaries), reflection (making sense of experience), action learning (project-based work to enhance learning in the context of business imperatives), and outdoor challenges (team-building exercises in outdoor or wilderness settings). (Day and Halpin, 2001, p. vii)

Most best-practice programs go beyond the traditional classroom format to include any or all of the following: stretch assignments or details to leadership positions, short-term projects overseen by preceptors, 360-degree or other rigorous types of assessment and feedback, mentoring or coaching, personal development plans, and structured reflection. Organizations in Day and Halpin's study believed that job assignments were particularly helpful to managers in learning about building teams,

---

[6] The military generally distinguishes between training (short-term skill development aimed at specific assignment needs) and education (conceptual knowledge with long-term career value).

how to be better strategic thinkers, and how to gain valuable persuasion and influence skills. Coaching, generally a relatively short-term activity done by external consultants, may be used to improve individual performance, enhance a career, or work through organizational issues such as change initiatives (Day and Halpin, 2001).

Day and Halpin (2001, p. vii) also point out that

> [t]he best-practice organizations find ways to integrate these various techniques of leadership development in making their initiatives holistic and systemic in nature. Effective leadership development appears to be a function of the interdependence of the various practices rather than a collection of independent programs. Finally, it is not necessarily a "best practice" that leads to successful development of leadership; rather it is the consistent implementation of any leadership development practice.

Military leader professional development is an accumulation of many experiences throughout one's career, including a range of duty assignments and educational preparation, both formal and self-directed. In response to the *CJCS Vision for Joint Officer Development* (U.S. Joint Chiefs of Staff, 2005), which outlines a learning continuum to develop officers with the skills, competencies, and experiences of a joint leader, each service is revising its community's career paths and educational curricula to adhere more closely to this model (U.S. Joint Chiefs of Staff, 2005, pp. 4–7). Structured job assignments and experiences can help officers grow as managers and leaders; for example, deployments may encourage a steeper rate of growth of leadership and management knowledge and skills, and perhaps enterprise knowledge and skills, through acculturation and in-depth experience. In addition, leader development can be fostered through explicit or implicit mentoring by senior staff and directed career counseling. All officers receive at least some career counseling that allows them to consider a range of career paths, including clinical, academic, or command or leadership. A critical part of leader development may also be an assessment of and feedback on the individual's strengths and weaknesses and the provision of advice on how best to build on the one and address the other. This can be approached through annual evaluations (discussed later) and the mentoring and career counseling process.

Incentives for individuals to apply for and remain in leadership positions could include the chance of being promoted or assigned to a more prestigious position, additional pay, performance bonuses, and nonpecuniary rewards, such as prestige and recognition. Generally, these rewards are grounded in comprehensive periodic evaluations of the individual's performance. Individuals could be evaluated on measurable and nonmeasurable indicators (including leader competencies) and asked to demonstrate how they contribute to and further organizational goals and missions.

Outcome

As noted earlier, the leader development process is designed to produce individuals who are qualified for executive-level positions and who possess the necessary skills, knowledge, and experience to perform successfully in these positions within the organizational context. Whether or not the outcome meets the expectations of the organization depends critically on the organization's approach to leader development and how well this approach is implemented and set within the organizational context and environment.

Data and Methods

To address the research questions listed in Chapter One, we used a variety of data-collection methods, including (1) a review of current materials from the services on leader development and career stages and (2) interviews with selected samples of military health care leaders and community managers, leaders of civilian health care organizations, and senior VHA leaders. We discuss these methods in the remainder of this chapter.

Review of Service Documents on Current Leader Development

We reviewed services' websites and other literature to understand how military medical leaders are currently developed in terms of the education and training that are required or desired at various points in one's career, as well as the typical career path of medical leaders in the different services and corps.[7]

Interviews

Military Health Professions Officers and Community Managers. We conducted interviews with 57 military leaders across the three services and with community managers from the various corps in each service. We selected a purposive sample of interviewees—senior leaders at the MTFs and community managers—to ensure some representation by corps within each service.

To select the sample of senior MTF leaders, we obtained a list of all the MTFs and sorted them by service and size (using the standardized workload measure reported by the Medical Expense and Performance Reporting System, the standard cost-accounting system used by the MHS). We then used information from the websites of the 20 largest facilities to determine who the commander and second-in-command were and to which corps they belonged. In this manner, we selected ten to 12 leaders who represented the various corps. At some of the larger facilities, in the first round of inter-

---

[7] As discussed in Chapter One, medical personnel are organized into different corps depending on their duties. For example, physicians are members of the MC. Across the services, health professions officers serve in the MC, DC, Army VC, NC, MSC, Army SP, and Air Force BSC.

views, we sought to interview the chief of staff or an HR representative. We solicited the help of the flag officer steering committee overseeing establishment of the joint medical education and training campus at Fort Sam Houston, Texas, in obtaining access to the selected sample. We were successful in obtaining interviews with all but two respondents. These interviews were generally hour-long telephone or in-person interviews. Interviews were guided by semistructured protocols, allowing us to collect similar information from each respondent but also providing the flexibility to ask more in-depth questions where appropriate.

We asked for assistance from the executive integrated process team in identifying corps community managers and in setting up the interviews. These managers were asked about both general career development of officers belonging to that community and their own careers, leader development opportunities, and support provided by the services.

Table 2.2 shows the distribution of respondents by corps and service. Not surprisingly, given that we targeted heads of MTFs, our sample is dominated by MC officers, although the sample does have a fair number of MSC (particularly in the case of the Army) and NC officers. Although we identify the respondents by their corps, as noted earlier, some headed workforce development and/or planning across the various communities and were able to speak about the career path and professional development of several corps, not just their own. Because this was a purposive sample, the analysis reported in later chapters may not represent the views of the larger population. However, these individuals were deliberately chosen because they were leading large MTFs and were a mix of O-6 and flag-rank officers—the group that was the focus of our study. The consistency of findings within and across the services suggests that the views of this expert sample provide valid, useful, and thoughtful perspectives on how the military leader development process works in practice and its perceived strengths and shortcomings.

Leaders of Civilian Health Care Organizations. To understand how civilian health care organizations identify, develop, and support leaders for executive positions, we undertook a series of interviews with 30 selected health care executives of nationally recognized health care systems and leaders of professional associations serving health care leaders. We sought to interview senior leadership at all the hospitals in our sample, defined as an executive leader (chief executive officer [CEO], chief operating officer [COO], chief medical officer, or chief nursing officer [CNO]), a ranking leader in the HR department, or an individual in charge of organizational development. We selected a deliberate sample of health care organizations in the private sector that were most likely to offer lessons learned for DoD. Our interviews were conducted in two phases—Phase I and Phase II—that covered the calendar years 2007 and 2008, respectively. The full sample is shown in Table 2.3.

Table 2.2
Interview Sample of Military Health Care Leaders,
by Service and Corps

Service and Corps	Number of Respondents
Army	
Medical	10
Dental	1
Nurse	3
Medical Service	8
Medical Specialist	2
Veterinary	1
Total	25
Navy	
Medical	7
Dental	1
Nurse	3
Medical Service	4
Total	15
Air Force	
Medical	7
Dental	1
Nurse	5
Medical Service	4
Biomedical Sciences	0
Total	17
Total, all services	57

Phase I Sample. The Phase I sample included three types of institutions—nonprofit hospitals, other types of hospitals, and professional associations. We wanted to identify top-performing hospitals to learn about best practices in leader development. To do so, we used two sets of rankings to select the sample for nonprofit hospitals. To be selected, an organization had to be identified in both sets of rankings. The first, the *U.S. News and World Report* annual ranking of U.S. hospitals, uses a variety of

Table 2.3
Interview Sample of Civilian Health Care Organizations, by Type and Phase of Study

Phase	Organization
Hospitals	
Phase I (2007)	Riverside Methodist Hospital
	Yale–New Haven Hospital
	Vanderbilt University Medical Center
	University of Michigan Hospitals and Health Centers
	Brigham and Women's Hospital
	University Hospitals Case Medical Center
	Charles F. Kettering Memorial Hospital
	Lancaster General Hospital
	Beth Israel Deaconess Medical Center
	University of Wisconsin Hospital and Clinics
	University of Kentucky Hospital
	William Beaumont Hospital–Troy
	Hospital Corporation of America
	Kaiser Permanente
Phase II (2008)	Cleveland Clinic
	Mayo Clinic
	Palo Alto Medical Foundation
	Henry Ford Hospital
	Virginia Mason
	Kaiser Foundation Health Plan and Hospitals
	Cedars Sinai Medical Center
	Trinity Health
Professional associations	
Phase I (2007)	American College of Healthcare Executives
	American College of Physician Executives
	American Organization of Nurse Executives

indicators to rank nonprofit hospitals, and reputation of excellence is among the most heavily weighted factors. To be eligible for inclusion in our sample, a hospital had to have at least one medical specialty ranked in the 2006 rankings. The second set of rankings was the Solucient Top 100 Hospitals list (now the Thomson Reuters Top 100 Hospitals Program), which identifies top-performing hospitals based on performance measures centered on clinical excellence, operating efficiency and financial health, and responsiveness to the community. Appendix A provides further details on the methodology used in both sets of rankings. Fifteen hospitals met the above-mentioned criteria. Three organizations refused to or did not respond to our request to participate in this study, leaving a total of 12 hospitals in our final sample, as shown in Table 2.3. Many of them are academic medical centers, which account for a small fraction of MTFs in the DoD system.

We also targeted large national hospital chains, including for-profit institutions and an integrated managed care organization.[8] The Hospital Corporation of America (HCA) is a for-profit hospital chain comprising locally managed facilities that included 170 hospitals and 113 outpatient centers in 20 states and employed approximately 180,000 people in 2006 (see HCA, undated, for current statistics). Kaiser Permanente is an integrated managed care organization that encompasses health plans, hospitals, and medical groups. As of 2006, Kaiser had a presence in nine states and is reported to be the largest managed care organization in the nation. Kaiser has nearly 150,000 employees, 37 medical centers, and 400 medical offices (see Kaiser Permanente, undated, for current statistics).

We identified three professional associations as most relevant for this study. These three associations have a collective membership of nearly 50,000 health care executives (including military health professions officers) and are very knowledgeable about the professional and leader development needs of the professions they represent in the health care industry. Moreover, all three offer some type of education or training focused on executive and leader development:

- The American College of Healthcare Executives (ACHE) is an international professional society of more than 30,000 health care executives who lead hospitals, health care systems, and other health care organizations (ACHE, undated).
- The American College of Physician Executives (ACPE) is an international association with more than 10,000 members in the United States and 33 other countries (ACPE, undated).
- The American Organization of Nurse Executives (AONE) is a national organization of more than 7,000 nurse leaders who design, facilitate, and manage care (AONE, undated).

---

[8] Despite repeated attempts, we were unable to secure participation from representatives at one additional for-profit hospital chain.

Phase II Sample. In 2008, we sought to expand the sample to include eight additional hospital systems that either had organizational structures more similar to those encountered in military treatment facilities, were physician-led, or were recognized for implementing leader development programs. Thus, we added three integrated group practices (Mayo Clinic, Cleveland Clinic, and Palo Alto Medical Foundation), along with Kaiser Foundation Health Plan and Hospitals, an integrated delivery system in which the payer and provider are one. We also added a handful of institutions actively implementing quality improvement processes and with highly regarded leadership development programs (Virginia Mason, Cedars Sinai Medical Center, Henry Ford Hospital, and Trinity Health). Several of these organizations were also physician-led (e.g., Mayo, Cleveland).

Total Interviews. In total, we interviewed 30 individuals across 25 organizations. In Phase I, we conducted 22 interviews across 17 organizations, including 17 interviews with leaders from the 12 nonprofit hospitals. Of the participating nonprofit organizations, there were five in which we interviewed both an executive and an HR senior leader. Among the other five organizations, we completed interviews with one executive from HCA (senior executive) and from Kaiser (physician-in-chief at one of Kaiser's medical facilities), as well as one executive from each of the three professional associations. In Phase II, we conducted interviews with one current or former top-level executive in each of the eight sampled organizations, for a total of eight interviews.

VHA Case Study. In addition to the private-sector interviews, we examined public health care systems—the PHS and the VHA—to understand how they developed and supported their leaders. The three senior PHS respondents noted that because their mission and staffing differed from that of the military, lessons learned from the PHS would be of limited relevance for our purposes. Thus, we eliminated the PHS as a source of data for our study.

The VHA, on the other hand, is similar in size and mission to DoD and falls under a cabinet-level official. Indeed, it is the most comparable organization to the MHS. Also, like DoD, it has made a serious commitment to strategic human capital development. The VHA has deliberately attempted to position itself as a learning organization dedicated to the education and development of all its employees, with formal processes in place to identify high-potential performers, to offer them systematic and carefully structured development and training opportunities, and to evaluate them against desired competencies. As such, we focused our efforts on the VHA and conducted 16 interviews with senior leaders at the VHA Central Office (VHACO) and with network and facility directors. These hour-long interviews were conducted by telephone or in person using a semistructured protocol. Table 2.4 shows the sample of respondents for the VHA interviews. Although a third of the sample consisted of facility and network directors (similar to the commanders of the MTFs), the sample

Table 2.4
Interview Sample of VHA Leaders, by Type

Type	Number of Respondents
Central office	11
Network and facility directors	5
Total	16

was heavily weighted in favor of those heading various offices responsible for leader development, employee education, workforce management, and organizational development, among others. The primary reason was that we needed to understand more fully the VHA's system of identifying, supporting, developing, and evaluating leaders. These interviews offered valuable lessons learned about both the process and implementation of a structured policy of leader and employee development.

However, our analysis of the VHA went well beyond interviews. We also researched its recent history, since it has transformed itself into a government health system that compares very favorably with private organizations. A large part of that transformation stemmed from its leader development program. Therefore, in addition to the interviews, we reviewed the extensive material the VHA provided on how it selects, develops, and provides incentives to its workforce.

Analytic Methods

As mentioned, we used a semistructured protocol for our interviews. This ensured that respondents were asked a common set of questions organized around the conceptual framework, but it also allowed for some latitude with respect to follow-up questions. Interviewees were asked for the following information:

- organizational environment and expectations (i.e., how they define an ideal leader, competencies and criteria used, changes in organizational context that might affect the kinds of skills leaders need)
- talent recruitment and management (i.e., methods used to recruit and identify potential leaders, career paths, succession planning, hiring from within and without)
- personnel evaluation protocols (i.e., metrics used for evaluation, organizational incentives)
- professional development activities (including job assignments and rotations, education and training, mentoring, career counseling, and feedback)
- challenges and lessons learned about effective leader development
- additional related comments.

In particular, we asked our military respondents what advice they might have for improving the current system of leader development. Given the emphasis on developing joint leaders, we also probed military respondents about the need for and feasibility of mandating joint professional education and experience for health professions officers.

Using the conceptual framework to define various coding "bins," or categories, we analyzed the data from our interview notes and transcripts, along with other documentation provided to us by respondents or that we collected about these institutions (e.g., from books or journal articles). In particular, we outlined broad themes that emerged from the separate analyses of the service interviews and then met as a team to conduct the cross-case analysis, in which each service was treated as the "unit of analysis." We grouped data from the three services by bin to look for patterns across the cases. This allowed us to come up with overarching themes that cut across services as well as themes that were unique to a service. The civilian interviews were coded as a separate case but under similar bins to allow us to draw out similarities and differences between the civilian and the military sectors. Unlike the other two sets of interviews, the VHA interviews and materials were more factually oriented and were analyzed to provide a descriptive understanding of the rationale for the model adopted by the VHA and the process of implementation while still adhering to the overall framework.

Along with our analysis, we examined the advice provided by our respondents about improving leader development in the military and looked for broad areas of consensus that could form the basis for recommendations.

Two caveats must be kept in mind. First, our samples of respondents from the military, civilian, and public sectors were expert samples, purposely chosen from the group of senior executives leading large organizations or facilities (the focus of our study) and not randomly selected. As such, they represent the views of our sample and cannot be generalized to the overall population.

Second, we accepted at face value what respondents told us about the perceived effectiveness of various leader development practices or competency frameworks. Thus, readers should keep in mind that the findings here—although they meet the test of logical reasonableness—are based on perceptions of respondents. However, previous literature has pointed to many of the strategies identified here as best practices, not simply in the health care field but also more broadly across the civilian sector.

Despite these two limitations, the results of this research make important contributions to understanding leader development practices in civilian and military health care organizations. Data from our interviews, as well as the extensive review of service documents and the literature, provide a rich portrait of how health care leaders are currently developed, the competencies required to be a successful leader in today's environment, perceived gaps in leader development, and some perceived best practices.

A Note on Terminology

Throughout this monograph, where we cite responses from those we interviewed, we use the following terminology to characterize the numbers of respondents associated with a particular response: few = one or two; some = three or four; several = five to ten; many = almost all of those interviewed; and mixed = no consensus, i.e., fewer than half of those interviewed supported one view.

CHAPTER THREE

How Military Health Care Leaders Are Currently Developed in the Services

The officer corps of the Army, Navy, and Air Force are composed of a diverse mix of grades or ranks, experience in terms of years of service, and occupations. Typically, those officers (in what are called "line" communities) enter, are developed, and advance differently from officers in the professions, such as doctors, dentists, and lawyers.[1] This chapter briefly discusses line officer career management but concentrates on career management and outcomes for health professions officers and profiles typical career paths. It is not intended to be comprehensive but, rather, is meant to be broadly descriptive of management practices across the three military services, and it provides an organizational and procedural context for the interviews discussed in the next chapter. Its intent is to contrast the patterns of officer service in the different occupations as a basis for understanding the more detailed analysis of how military health care officers perceive themselves to be developed and supported.[2]

Military officer personnel management can be generally described as a life-cycle model within a closed overall system. The life cycle follows a progression of entry, development (training, education, and experience through assignments), rewards (compensation and promotion), and transition (separating or retiring). *Closed system* means that all entry is as an O-1 at the beginning of a career, with little to no lateral entry at later points in a career profile.

Each service provides life-cycle models as career guides for officers. For example, the Air Force career path guide is shown as a pyramid with lieutenants at the base and colonels at the apex. The pyramid is carved horizontally into grade bands (e.g., captain and major/lieutenant colonel) that show expected development, education and train-

---

[1] While each service takes a slightly different approach to categorizing occupations, the line communities include such occupations as infantry, pilots, surface warfare officers, and more specialized occupations, including intelligence, communications, and operations research. Occupations are managed as competitive categories; groups of officers compete among themselves for developmental opportunities and promotions. Each service is different in this regard, with the Navy making the most use of separate competitive categories and the Army and Air Force placing more officers in fewer categories. The health services occupations, for the most part, are each a separate competitive category.

[2] See service documents such as Headquarters, U.S. Department of the Army (2010) or Air Force Instruction 36-2640 (2008) for more complete descriptions.

ing, and assignments at each level. The Army model is a rectangle with vertical sections for the different ranks. For each rank, expected professional military education (PME), additional training, typical assignments, and self-development requirements are shown. There is a separate model for each Army branch (e.g., Infantry, Armor).

While generally using this life-cycle model of officer management, the health professions officer occupations differ somewhat in that some hew closely to the model (i.e., MSC); some follow a different model, particularly with respect to entering and rewarding (i.e., MC and DC); and some fall between the two extremes (i.e., NC). This chapter illustrates officer management practices for the health professions officer occupations or corps.

A detailed description of the typical assignment and educational opportunities for line and health professions officers can be found in Appendix B.

Life-Cycle Model for Health Professions Officers

While the health professions generally follow the life-cycle models described in the beginning of this chapter, they differ significantly from line communities, particularly for some corps, such as medical. Specifically, there are marked differences in the requirements regarding joint education and experience for promotion to flag rank. As such, we discuss these requirements in a separate section.

Entering

Compared with the line communities, there are many more ways to enter the military as a commissioned officer. For example, the Army lists, in addition to the traditional sources (such as the military academy, the Reserve Officers' Training Corps [ROTC], and Officer Candidate School), the following sources for "non–due course" officers:[3] U.S. Army Recruiting Command programs, Health Profession Scholarship Program, Financial Assistance Program, Civilian Education Delay, direct accessions fully qualified and licensed in their respective specialties, reserve or National Guard accession to active duty, voluntary and involuntary branch transfers, and interservice transfers. For physicians, the Armed Forces Health Professions Scholarship Program and the Uniformed Services University of Health Sciences are the two primary sources for the Army and Navy, with about 77 percent and 15 percent, respectively, represented from each service. More than 95 percent of Air Force entering physicians are direct accessions, according to Defense Manpower Data Center statistics for FY 2008. Moreover,

---

[3] The term refers to officers who are commissioned at a higher rank because they have an advanced degree. The Army defines a due course officer as one who has been on continuous active duty since commissioning as a second lieutenant and who has neither failed selection for promotion nor been selected for promotion from below the zone.

a physician or dentist is not constrained by the requirement that he or she be able to complete 20 years of active commissioned service by age 62.

The key to understanding different entry sources and practices is the concept of constructive credit for advanced education, special experience, or prior commissioned service. Constructive service credit

> provides a person who begins commissioned service after obtaining the additional education, training, or experience required for appointment . . . as an officer in a health profession, with a grade and date of rank comparable to that attained by officers who begin commissioned service after getting a baccalaureate degree and serve for the period of time it would take to obtain the additional education. (DoDI 6000.13, 1997, para. 6.1.2)

So, for example, credit of health professions other than medicine and dentistry could be for up to two years for a master's degree and up to four years for a doctorate. Also, credit of one-half year for each year of experience, up to a maximum of three years of constructive credit, may be granted. The total entry grade credit granted can be no more than that required for an officer to be eligible for an original appointment in the grade of major or lieutenant commander. However, Title 10 of the U.S. Code allows for original appointments for qualified doctors of medicine, osteopathy, or dentistry to be made in the grades of first lieutenant or lieutenant junior grade through colonel or Navy captain. Each service secretary can choose how to implement these sections of law and policy.

As a result, health professions officers may enter as lieutenants or ensigns and follow a path not unlike that of a line officer or enter at a higher grade or rank. These latter officers have the required health professions education and experience but not the military experience that line officers of a similar rank would have.

Developing

Health professions officers are subject to the same training requirements for skills, knowledge, and attributes as every other officer, but the early focus is on the domain or functional knowledge and practices of their specialty. Other training and education requirements might apply to officers in a particular corps. However, officers who enter at advanced grades (O-3 and above) with constructive credit forgo many early developmental opportunities typically experienced by junior officers. For these officers, experience is missed or compressed compared with officers who enter without constructive credit. In general, health professions officers follow the services' educational model of entry-officer education, intermediate-level education, and senior service college. For example, the Air Force cautions that officers who have not completed PME within a reasonable time after they become eligible will not be very competitive for upward-mobility jobs. As a result, officers are encouraged to attend intermediate service and senior service school by correspondence or seminar rather than in residence.

Moreover, health professions officers usually have more restricted opportunities for in-residence attendance at some institutions, such as the senior service colleges, where around 12 seats might be available each year. Besides PME, different corps and specialties within corps will have requirements for internship, residency and fellowship training, advanced degrees, and continuing education.

The opportunities for gaining experience through assignment depend on requirements and developmental needs. Typically, each service has tracks in which health professions officers will primarily develop. They could differ by corps and might include clinical, academic, research, administrative, staff, executive, or operational tracks. The patterns of gaining experience and the emphasis on solid performance in assignments are similar to those of the line communities, as discussed previously. For example, the Army stresses for each of its corps, such as the DC, the need to have institutional training, operational assignments, and self-development at each junior and senior level of service and provides corresponding life-cycle development and utilization models. The processes are similar to those of the line communities as well. For example, the Air Force developmental team for nurses will review an officer's future potential in clinical, education and training, or executive leadership areas and make suggestions for moving into different tracks to broaden experience or gain more depth in a particular track. Also, as with the line communities, notional career paths give officers information about the types of positions available in the different tracks at different grade and experience levels. Examples of these career paths are shown in Figures 3.1 through 3.4. Figure 3.1 shows the career path for the Navy NC, Figures 3.2 and 3.3 for the Air Force NC, and Figure 3.4 for the Army NC.

Command is an important milestone for health professions officers, as it is for line officers. Most O-6 command positions in the Army and Navy are authorized for any qualified medical professional, and officers in all the corps aspire to them.[4] Central selection boards meet periodically to designate officers for particular commands.

For those officers who aspire to executive leadership in MTFs (i.e., as executive or commanding officers), Congress has mandated attainment of 39 competencies outlined in the JMESP, discussed in Chapter Two.

Joint Education and Experience

In the 2005 *Vision for Joint Officer Development*, then-Chairman of the Joint Chiefs of Staff Peter Pace emphasized the need for *all* colonels and Navy captains to be educated and experienced in joint matters (U.S. Joint Chiefs of Staff, 2005). Until recently, the way to develop joint officers has been to provide officers with the opportunity to attend schools offering JPME Phases I and II and to serve for specified periods in billets that provide them with joint duty experience. These billets constitute the Joint Duty

---

[4]   The Army refers to such positions as "branch immaterial," while the Navy uses the billet designator code "2000."

Figure 3.1
Navy Nurse Corps Career Path

	Operational	Clinical	Administration/2XXX	Education	Research
CAPT (EXECUTIVE)	Headquarters Staff; Advanced Practitioner Afloat; Mobilization; CO/XO FH; SNE–TAH, FH, OCONUS; Training (T): (16), (20), (21), (23)	Headquarters Staff; Program Manager; Clinical Director; Advanced Practitioner; Head, Command PI; CNS, MTF (large); Specialty Leader; T: (13), (14), (15), (16), (17), (18), (20), (21)	CO/XO MTF (small, med); CO/XO NMCL; SNE, MTF; Director, MTF (large); Headquarters SECNAV/OASD(HA); TRICARE Regional Offices; HSO Staff; T: (13), (14), (15), (16), (17), (18), (19), (20)	DEPCOM, NMETC; CO/XO NSHS; CO/XO MTF (small, med); Dept Head SEAT, MTF (large); Headquarters Staff; Program Manager; Specialty Leader; T: (14), (15), (16), (20)	Dir, Clinical Invest NMETC; Head, Clinical Invest MTF; Clinical Researcher, NSHS; Clinical Research, NAMRL; Nrsg Research Coord, MTF; Program Manager; Specialty Leader; T: (14), (16)
CDR (SENIOR)	Headquarters Staff; Advanced Practitioner Afloat; CRNA Afloat; Naval Doctrine Center; COMPHIGRUs; Senior Nurse–AH (crew); Specialty Leader; Mobilization: SNE–TAH, FH; Dept Head–TAH, FH, etc.; T: (5), (16), (20), (21), (22), (23)	Advanced Practitioner; CNS, MTF (large or med); Head, Command PI; Headquarters Staff; Program Manager; Specialty Leader; T: (5), (12), (13), (16), (17), (20), (21)	Headquarters Staff; OASD(HA); TRICARE Regional Offices; HSO Staff; SNE, MTF (small) or NMCL; Dept Head, MTF (med, small); Div Off, MTF (large); OIC, Branch Clinic; Senior Nurse, Branch Clinic; T: (5), (13), (16), (17), (19), (20), (22)	Headquarters Staff; Program Manager, NMETC; Program Manager, CNET; Deputy OIS; Dept Head SEAT, MTF (large); Dept Head SEAT, MTF (med); Academic Director, NSHS; T: DUINS, ETMS/EdD, (5), (16)	Head, Clinical Invest MTF; Nrsg Research Coord, MTF; Clinical Researcher, NSHS; Clinical Researcher, NAMRL; Specialty Leader; T: DUINS (PhD), (5), (16)
LCDR (INTERMEDIATE)	Advanced Practitioner Afloat; CRNA Afloat; COMPHIGRUs; Ship Nurse–CV/CVN; Staff Nurse–CRTS, FSSG, FST; Instructor–FHOTC; Mobilization; Div Off–TAH, –H; Staff Nurse–CRTS, FSSG, FST; T: DUINS, (3), (5), (7), (8), (9), (10), (11), (20)	Advanced Practitioner, MTF; CNS, MTF (large or med); T: DUINS (MSN, PhD, CRNA), (3), (5), (11), (12)	Dept Head, MTF OCONUS; Dept Head, MTF (small); Div Off, MTF OCONUS; Div Off, MTF (med); Senior Nurse, Branch Clinic; T: (3), (5), (12), (13), (20)	Headquarters Staff; Instructor "A" or "C" School; Instructor OIS; Dept Head SEAT, MTF (med); Dept Head SEAT, MTF (small); Div Off, SEAT, MTF; T: DUINS, ETMS, EdD, (3), (5), (10)	Nrsg Research Coord, MTF; Clinical Researcher, NAMRL; T: DUINS (PhD), (3), (5), (10)
LT (BASIC)	Staff Nurse–CRTS, FSSG, FST; Ship Nurse–CV/CVN; Instructor–FHOTC; Mobilization; Staff Nurse–TAH, FH, CRTS, FSSG, FST, etc.; T: (2), (4), (6), (7), (8), (9), (11)	Staff Nurse, MTF/Clinic; T: DUINS (MSN, CRNA), (2), (4), (6)	Div Off, MTF OCONUS; Div Off, MTF (small); T: DUINS (MSN, MBA, MPH), (2), (4)	Instructor "A" School; Staff SEAT, MTF; Staff OIS; T: (2), (4)	
LTJG/ENS	Mobilization: Staff Nurse for TAH, FH, CRTS, FSSG, FST, etc.; T: Mobilization and Platform Training, (1), (4), (6)	Staff Nurse, CONUS MTF, subspecialty and skill development; T: (1), (4), (6)	Staff Nurse, CONUS MTF, subspecialty and skill development; T: (1), (4), (6)	Staff Nurse, CONUS MTF, subspecialty and skill development; T: (1), (4), (6)	Staff Nurse, CONUS MTF, subspecialty and skill development; T: (1), (4), (6)

Left margin labels: CO XO SNE; Career Progression, Development and Specialization. Column-separating bands: Operational Readiness Training.

(1) Division Officer Course at OIS; (2) Intermed. Officers Leadership Training Course; (3) Adv. Officers Leadership Training Course; (4) Basic Medical Dept. Officer Course; (5) Adv. Medical Department Officer Course; (6) Intermed. Officers Leadership Training Course; (7) Critical Care Air Transport Course; (8) Flight Nurse School; (9) En Route Care Training; (10) Joint Operational Medical Management Course; (11) Navy Trauma Training Course; (12) Clinic Management Course; (13) TRICARE Fin. Mgt. Exec Course; (14) PXO and Command Leadership Training; (15) MHS Capstone Course; (16) Interagency Institute for FHCE; (17) JCAHO Fellowship; (18) Wharton Fellow Program; (19) Congressional Fellowship; (20) (Service) War College (Jr or Sr); (21) Indus. College of the Armed Forces; (22) Sr. Officers Course in Military Justice; (23) Joint Task Force Senior Medical Leadership Seminar

SOURCE: U.S. Department of the Navy, Bureau of Medicine and Surgery, 2005.

RAND MG967-3.1

Figure 3.2
Life-Cycle Model for Air Force Nurse Corps Career Path

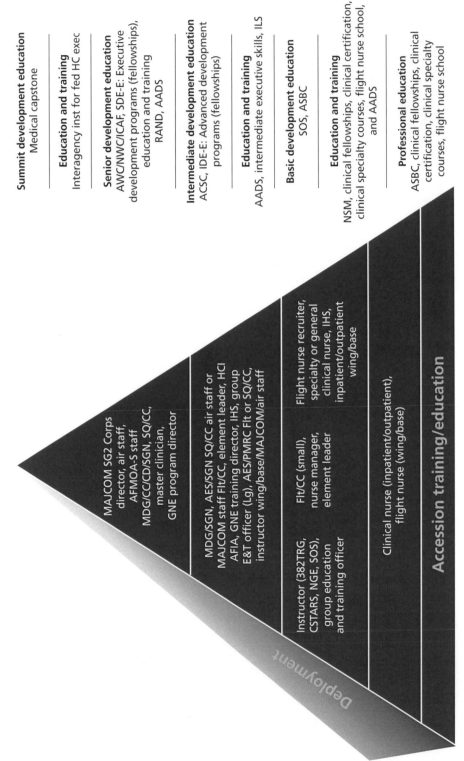

SOURCE: U.S. Air Force Medical Service.

RAND *MG967-3.2*

Figure 3.3
Air Force Nurse Corps Career Path

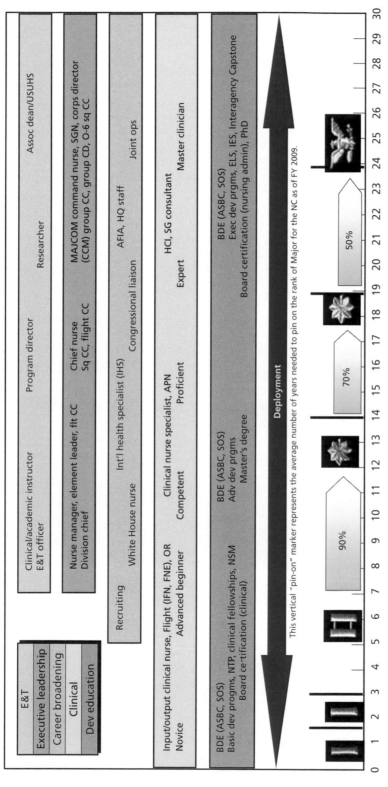

NOTE: The timeline bars illustrate potential developmental opportunities during an officer's career and can be used as a guideline for career planning. The promotion data on the lower portion of the page illustrates the average in-the-zone rates that last seven promotional boards. Some officers receive constructive credit for experience or education prior to their military service. The vertical "pin-on" markers indicated the average year for promotion and are calculated by taking the difference between an officer's date of rank for a grade and his or her total active military commissioned service data. The data are current as of FY 2009.

SOURCE: U.S. Air Force Medical Service.

RAND MG967-3.3

Figure 3.4
Army Nurse Corps Career Path

Years	0	5	10	15	20	25	30

Rank	LT 0–4	CPT 5–9	MAJ 9–15	LTC 16–21	COL 22–30		

Professional military education	BOLC	CCC		ILE		SSC	

Additional training

AOC/ASI course | Postgraduate education, TWI, Baylor HCA, fellowships, Interagency institute for Federal Health Care Executives

Army nurse preceptorship program | Head nurse leadership course | Advanced nurse leadership course | Executive skills course

CBRNE, BLS, PALS, ACLS TNCC, ATLS, CR, ABLS, TCMC, JOMCC, MMHAC, HLSMEC, TC3, ENCP, JECC, Div surg course, Primary flight surgeon course

Airborne, Air assault, EFMB

Typical assignments

Lieutenant/captain	Lieutenant/captain	Lieutenant/captain	Colonel
TDA Staff/charge nurse Preceptor Assistant head nurse Unit education coordinator ROTC counselor USAREC recruiter Company commander Nurse practitioner Nurse anesthetist **TOE** FORSCOM staff nurse	**TDA** Staff/head nurse Clinical nurse specialist Nurse practitioner Midwife Enlisted MOS instructor Director/deputy MOS course Team commander/USAREC Executive officer/USAREC **TOE** CSH head nurse FST chief nurse DMRTI instructor	**TDA** Staff/head nurse/MEDCEN Chief, section, ward, or clinic Assistance chief nurse, MEDDAC Chief nurse/DCN Director/deputy AOC/ASI course Nurse methods analyst Chief, informatics Chief, hospital education Consultant Branch-immaterial command **TOE** CSH assist CN DCDD/Combat development JRTC O/C JRCAB/DMSB	**TDA** Assistant chief nurse MAJCOM chief nurse DCN/chief nurse Brigade chief nurse Chief, section, department Chief, dept nursing science Director, anesthesia program Staff officer CIO, deputy CIO Chief, AN HRC Chief nurse, USAREC, ROTC Branch-immaterial command **TOE** CSH CN MC/MBDE CN FORSCOM CN

Self-development	Continuing health education
	Professional board certification

SOURCE: Headquarters, U.S. Department of the Army, 2007, p. 127.

RAND *MG967-3.4*

Assignment List (JDAL). The new DoD policy on joint officer management (DoDI 1300.19, 2010) acknowledges that joint duty experience may be gained in non-JDAL billets and that the level of joint experience attained by an officer is a function of the currency, frequency, and intensity of experience rather than an arbitrary length of time in a billet. The common requirement is that the appropriate level of JPME be completed to achieve joint qualification.

However, both the traditional and current DoD policies (DoDI 1300.20, 1996; DoDI 1300.19, 2010) preclude positions requiring officers in the professional specialties from being on the JDAL. In addition, professional officers and those in the technical and scientific specialties are provided with waivers on a case-by-case basis from the requirement that all officers being considered for promotion to general or flag officer have served in joint duty assignments. Health professions officers, particularly in some corps, have few positions they can fill in joint organizations and, as mentioned earlier, DoD policy has been to exclude medical and legal officers from serving on the JDAL. Of the 9,000 JDAL assignments, most focus on operations or institutional needs; few require health service qualifications or focus specifically on the MHS. See Kirby and Thie (2009) for a more complete assessment of health professions officers and joint qualifications.

Becoming fully joint-qualified requires both experience and education. Health professions officers have more limited opportunities for joint professional education and training when compared with nonmedical officers. For example, some communities in the medical departments (specifically MC officers) are not required to complete PME and JPME I in the usual prescribed time frames, largely because of the need to complete medical education and training related to professional medical credentialing during the same period. Thus, the JPME I requirement is often deferred for medical officers until they are promoted to the rank of lieutenant colonel or commander. In addition, medical departments in each service are offered very few seats at JPME II sites.

There are large opportunity costs in sending additional health professions officers, particularly highly trained clinicians, either to a resident JPME school for a sustained period or to work on joint matters for two to three years. There are other costs to be considered as well. Maintaining clinical skills requires continuing and extended practice. Sending clinicians away for long periods on joint duty assignments—which, by definition, are not clinical—is likely to have a significant adverse effect on their proficiency levels.

Incentivizing

Pay. Health professions officers are compensated using the same system as that for the line communities reviewed earlier. However, because health professionals have attractive and lucrative private-sector opportunities, they are offered additional compensation to stay in the military. The services thus use a series of recruitment and retention tools, including scholarship programs, accession bonuses, and special pays, to recruit and retain health care officers. For example, physicians, dentists, and certain nurses have such retention incentives as board-certified pay, variable special pay, incentive special pay, and retention bonuses. These pays vary based on years of service, years of obligation, or area of specialization "but in aggregate can supplement military pay by substantial amounts—for example, by more than $100,000 annually for some physicians" (DoD, 2008b, p. 72). Within the past year, special pays for other health professionals, such as licensed clinical psychologists, licensed clinical social workers, physician assistants, and licensed veterinary officers, have been authorized by Congress.

Promotion. The evaluation and promotion processes are similar to those for the line communities with some exceptions, primarily for physicians and dentists who are exempt from the controls mandated by Congress for grades O-4, O-5, and O-6. As a result, promotion planning for these two professions differs somewhat. For example, if the number of officers to be recommended for promotion equals the number to be considered, all fully qualified officers are also best qualified and thus could be selected. For officers who receive constructive credit at entry, consideration for promotion is based on the date of achievement of the current grade held. Thus, promotion opportunity tends to be higher for these two professions, and promotions tend to occur regularly at the sixth, 12th, and 18th anniversaries of entry. For example, in the Army, recent primary-zone selection rates for MC and DC O-6s have been above 80 percent, while line rates were around 53 percent and other health professions were below the line rate. These rates vary from year to year, but the pattern generally holds.

Transitioning

The separation and retirement system is similar to that of the line communities, with some exceptions. Accession incentives and certain retention incentives require specified periods of active-duty service before leaving is possible. Retirement is after the same minimum period of active-duty service and no later than age 62, as for line communities, but a service secretary may defer the retirement age of a physician, dentist, or nurse.

Grade and Year-of-Service Outcomes

This section shows typical outcomes by grade and year of service for a line community, MC, and NC. These outcomes are typical of all the services. In Figures 3.5 through 3.7, we show the percentage of officers in each community who are at a given year of service.

Figure 3.5 shows the grade and experience profile of a line community. Analysts typically represent these profiles as a smoothed representation of a desirable profile. The figure presents actual data for the end of FY 2008, so it shows some of the issues

Figure 3.5
Grade and Experience Outcomes for Line Community Officers, Representative of All Services, FY 2008

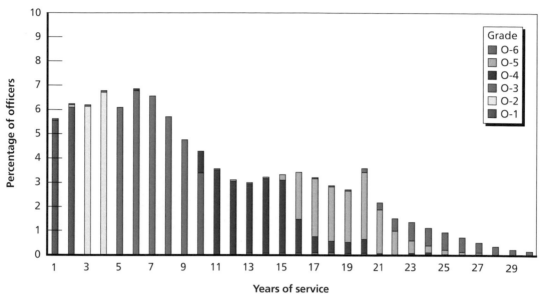

RAND *MG967-3.5*

Figure 3.6
Grade and Experience Outcomes for Medical Corps Officers, Representative of All Services, FY 2008

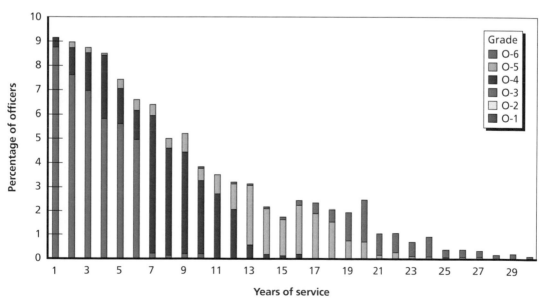

RAND *MG967-3.6*

Figure 3.7
Grade and Experience Outcomes for Nurse Corps Officers, Representative of All Services, FY 2008

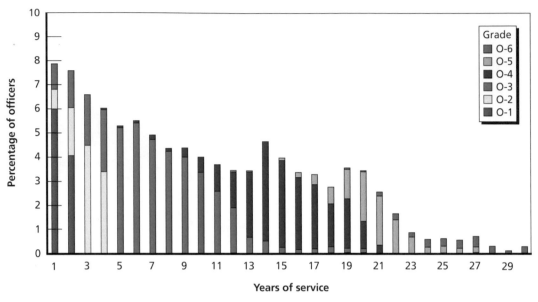

of managing officers within a closed system. For example, either different numbers of accessions or differing retention patterns in some years lead to the spikes in certain year-of-service groups. But, in general, the figure shows the distribution typical of a line community in term of grade and years of experience. This profile has somewhat higher-than-normal retention between four and eight years of service because of the high proportion of officers in certain communities with extended initial service requirements, but, after that, officers are making stay-or-go decisions. Also, captains or Navy lieutenants (O-3s) typically do not continue in service if they do not make an O-4 promotion, while majors and lieutenant commanders (O-4s) usually will continue to 20 years of service, with some selectively continuing to 24 years.

Figure 3.6 is a similar portrayal but for the MC. Some differences are easily seen. First, there are no lieutenants or ensigns. MC officers, as discussed earlier, enter at higher grades with constructive credit for education or experience. If they enter as O-3s, entry into the next higher grade (O-4) is four years sooner than it is for line officers, and it can be earlier than that. Compared to the line communities, proportionally more of MC officers are in the early years of service, and there are proportionally fewer at each year of service beyond around 14 years. Continuation beyond 20 years, the first retirement point, is lower than for the line community.

Figure 3.7 represents the NC profile. There are lieutenants and ensigns in the early years of service, as in the line communities, but also some O-3s who entered with constructive credit, as in the MC. There are proportionally more officers in early years of service than was seen in the line communities but fewer than in the MC; there are fewer proportionally in the higher grades than in either the line communities or the MC. Continuation after around 22 years of service drops precipitously, as in the MC.

This chapter provided a brief overview of the typical way in which health professions officers are managed in the services, their typical life cycles and career paths, and how they differ from those of line communities. This discussion sets the context for the next chapter, which presents findings from our interviews with military officers in which we asked about the current system for developing military health care leaders and their perceptions about its effectiveness.

CHAPTER FOUR

Findings from Interviews with Military Health Care Leaders: A Cross-Case Analysis

In this chapter, we present overarching themes that we identified from our cross-case analysis of interviews with 57 leaders from the three services, conducted during 2007 and 2008.[1] Appendixes C through E present findings from the Army, Navy, and Air Force interviews separately. Following the conceptual framework described in Chapter Two, we organized the key findings under the following broad areas: (1) context, organizational environment, and organizational leader expectations; (2) approach to leader development (i.e., how to select, how to develop, and how to incentivize); and (3) outcome in terms of whether the individuals produced by the system have the knowledge, skills, and abilities needed to perform successfully as senior medical leaders.[2]

Note that we refer to all respondents in a gender-neutral way to ensure anonymity, but our sample included men and women.

Context, Organizational Environment, and Organizational Leader Expectations

Context and Organizational Environment

Several respondents recognized the complexity of the military environment and its effects on leader expectations.

Particularly among Army and Navy respondents, leaders noted that the military and their particular service have become quite complex on a number of levels. First, leaders in the Army and Navy commented on the challenges of *managing a workforce* that now includes military, civilian, and contract workers. According to these respon-

---

[1] As defined earlier, in the cross-case analysis, each service was a "case." We combined data across the services within each coding category to identify themes and issues common to all services, as well those that appeared to be specific to an individual service.

[2] As noted earlier, throughout this monograph, where we cite responses from those we interviewed, we use the following terminology to characterize the number of respondents associated with a particular response: few = one or two; some = three or four; several = five to ten; many = almost all of those interviewed; and mixed = no consensus, i.e., fewer than half of those interviewed supported one view.

dents, this diversity creates an environment in which individuals are working under different rules, goals, procedures, and expectations. One Navy commander described their MTF as a "fragmented organization" and noted the challenges of leading in this context:

> You're dealing with three different systems. Often, you have military, civilian[s], and contractors, all of whom have different rules, have different goals, have different personnel structures and plans. And so, yes, these become much more fragmented than they used to be. And I think that's clearly an issue. . . . There's this larger turnover [with contractors]. You have little control.

Second, some leaders identified ways in which the *demands of war* affect leaders and leader development. For example, a few Army leaders reported that the ongoing wars have influenced expectations for leaders, who now need to know how to handle the effects of the "stresses of war" on those they supervise and their families. For example, one Army respondent believed that persistent war has dramatically changed the skills demanded of leaders:

> I think today, because we're at war, it's more important that we be engaged and get down and talk to them [supervisees] about their families. . . . What I have found over the last two years and in this job is that engaged leadership makes a big difference. I send out emails periodically to tell them what's going on. . . . Those are the types of things that I think because of the war and people are working long hours, we're deploying soldiers, stress on families, all of those things are important. And it's different than ten years ago. We've been in this war, what . . . five, almost six years now? So you have to look at it from what is the environment and what are the skill sets that we need?

Other leaders commented on the ways in which deployments created churn in MTFs and placed further strains on leaders. According to one Navy leader, deployments have created an incentive to staff certain positions with civilians to provide stability and "corporate continuity in product lines." However, several other Navy respondents cited potentially negative consequences of the new staffing arrangements. In one MTF, deployments had left a very limited number of civil service employees to supervise contract workers. The large numbers of civilian workers in another MTF also adversely affected the remaining military workers, who had to work harder and take on military-specific collateral duties (e.g., serving on committees).

Finally, a few leaders in the Navy identified new productivity demands that are shaping what is expected of leaders, who is selected, and how they are evaluated. These respondents noted that, unlike in years past when medical officers were judged on how well they supported the force and their families, there has been a decade-long movement to evaluate medical leaders more on "the bottom line" and their contributions to productivity. As one commander explained,

> You have to understand the business of medicine now. It's crucial, because we were never judged before on our ability to bring a product in—product per dollar. That was never in the mix. You were only judged by [what you] did [to] support the operational fighting forces. Did you take safe care of the families that were entrusted to you? . . . They didn't care how many patients you saw, how many patients you didn't see, as long as the care was safe, and it was satisfying—and that the wartime fighters had no complaints. . . . But what's changed in the last ten years is that you can't survive now in running a medium- to big-sized military treatment facility unless you understand the business of medicine.

Respondents in all three services identified differences in opportunities for leadership and growth across the corps.

Several leaders in the Army and Navy believed that, when compared to MSC officers, MC officers are at a disadvantage in obtaining leadership skills. Some of these respondents believed that because of the length of time required for clinical training and the demand to keep such officers in clinical positions, it often takes longer and is more difficult for MC providers to gain the requisite skills and advance to leadership positions. In the Army, several leaders reported that MSC officers gain leadership experience faster than MC officers. One Army physician identified a tension in decision-making about how to address this issue:

> Medical Service Corps officers, on the other hand, have a lot more opportunity to command. Rarely do you have a Medical Corps officer who can command a company. Often, the first time that a Medical Corps officer can command is at a clinic level or rarely at a fort surgical team level. . . . That's a big shortfall, but how do you fix that? By taking physicians out of their clinical practice and putting them in command?

Other leaders in the various services pointed to particular corps that were perceived to have limited opportunities for advancement and growth. For example, several Navy respondents reported that NC officers often do not get executive-level leadership opportunities until later in their careers, and, as a result, one noted, post-command options are very limited. One Navy leader explained that because dentists are in short supply, it is difficult to send them to leadership training. An Army leader observed that SP officers are unfairly limited in their ability to attain command positions because their corps does not have deputy command positions and, under the policy of branch-immaterial commands, must compete against other corps (MSC, MC, NC) officers coming out of deputy command positions. This leader argued, "We should be afforded the opportunity just like the other five corps, to be able to broaden our experience and grow the best officers, because we have some extremely fine officers that have been overlooked."

In the Air Force, some leaders noted that command of bedded facilities is reserved for physicians, which affected leadership opportunities for MSC officers.[3] One respondent believed that this decision exacerbated the problem of retention among MSC officers, stating that a number of MSC officers were demoralized by

> the decision by the Surgeon General that only physicians can command bedded facilities. Many people made a decision about the terminus of their career based on that decision.

Another Air Force leader identified a lack of leadership opportunities for BSC officers.

Some respondents commented on the systems for selection and competition for rank, revealing differences across the services in a model of "best in breed" versus "best in show" and their influence on leadership.

Characterizing it as a system of "best in breed" rather than "best in show," all Air Force respondents described the competition for rank as one conducted within corps and not across corps. A few respondents thought this system had a direct influence on the type of leaders selected (see the section "Outcome," later in this chapter).

Several Army respondents commented on the designation of most command positions as branch-immaterial, and many believed it was a fair policy because it allowed those with strong records to rise above others. However, as noted earlier, one leader believed that SP officers were adversely affected by this policy.

Some respondents noted that rank does not equate to leadership.

In the Air Force, several leaders noted different processes for promotion and determining rank in the medical and line communities, in which rank equates to leadership in the line community but not for medical officers. As one respondent explained,

> The Medical Corps and Dental Corps tend to use promotion opportunity as a retention and recruiting tool. And so we have a lot of full colonels that are not necessarily good leaders. They're great clinicians, and that's what we're paying them for, and that's what we want to keep them for. But they're not necessarily good leaders. On the line side, the line cannot understand how you can have so many O-6s who aren't leaders. But that really is the distinction on the line side. It truly is a pyramid. Within the medics, we admittedly promote more than we should if it [is] based solely on leadership. So rank and leadership do not always correlate.

---

[3] A "bedded facility" is one with hospital beds providing for longer periods of care, as opposed to an outpatient clinic, which has beds only for short-term stays, such as postoperative recovery.

Navy respondents also commented on the relationship between rank and leadership. A few believed that a "rank-conscious" culture limited the Navy's ability to identify and groom talent. One leader noted,

> We do tend at times to be very rank-conscious and reticent to step outside of that structure and say, . . . "I'm going to name this O-3 to be the division head over these O-4s because I think [he or she is] a better performer."

Similarly, another commander believed that the biggest challenge the Navy faces in identifying and supporting high-potential officers is "being stuck in the way they've always done it." Others were even more critical, noting that the Navy's "lock-step" requirement that an individual needed to be a director, then an executive officer (XO), then a commanding officer (CO) overlooks other opportunities for individuals to develop skills, demonstrate their potential, and be selected, thus resulting in the loss of leaders with great potential. One leader stated,

> We get so locked into [the] department head/director/XO/CO [route] . . . we oftentimes don't see these other opportunities . . . that help not only develop those skills, but also help the individual demonstrate [his or her] ability.

Retention problems were seen as inhibiting leader development.

Across the services, leaders reported that poor retention adversely affected the military's ability to develop leaders. Some believed that it limited the availability of mentors for younger leaders. Others noted that losing quality individuals translates to a loss of future quality leaders. "There's a lot of people that have left the Army that would have been great leaders because the opportunities are different on the outside," said one Army leader.

Several leaders identified contributing factors, such as the inability to offer financial incentives or higher salaries to compete with civilian organizations, as well as deployment duration. Some also believed that family issues and concerns about lifestyle changes served as a significant barrier to leader recruitment and development.

Organizational Expectations for Leaders

Although most respondents were asked in our interviews how their particular service defined an ideal leader, many responded by providing their opinions about what they felt were important characteristics or criteria for leaders.

Many respondents believed that experience was a critical criterion for leaders—particularly experience in a broad set of assignments.

Across the services, many respondents stressed that leaders needed to be "well rounded," have a variety of assignments that gave them broad exposure to a variety of jobs and settings, and demonstrate success in leading at these lower levels and gaining positions of increasing responsibility. For example, one Navy respondent argued that leaders needed "experience in doing something similar at a smaller command. . . . Something that would have exposed them to all the intricacies of managing a medical center." Similarly, one Air Force leader explained, "To really develop somebody's skill set and an understanding of our system, they really need to be moving around and understanding why MacDill is different from Altus, and it's different from Grand Forks and Yokota in Japan." Many respondents across the services also believed that the breadth of experience should include experience in warfighting and a "worthy deployment history."

"Soft" and "hard" leadership skills were seen as a necessity by many leaders.

In terms of soft skills, many respondents across the services considered "interpersonal skills" and "people skills" important for military medical leaders. Some characterized these as "intangible" and "less didactic or technical" and included in this skill set the abilities to work as part of a team, build strong teams, mentor and develop subordinates (e.g., act like a "good parent," "empowering them to be able to do what they need to do"), create positive climates that "people can grow in," listen to subordinates' concerns, inspire and acknowledge contributions of others, and create consensus. One Army leader explained,

> I would expect the Army to place high value on those of us who are able to apply the soft skills across an organization, and be able to coach, teach, mentor, and motivate vastly different groups of people within our organization. . . . It is not enough to know the regs, know the rules, be able to write an operation order; that is simply not enough. You've got to be able to read people, interact with people, manage large groups of diverse people.

Similarly, an Air Force respondent commented, "Interpersonal skills have been key . . . because a lot of it is not what you do individually but how well you inspire and you influence others to achieve those organizational objectives."

Many of these same leaders also highlighted the value of communication skills. One Air Force respondent stated, "I think the single greatest determinant of a leader, military or civilian, is their ability to communicate verbally and in writing." Similarly, when asked what to look for in identifying potential leaders, an Army leader responded, "Bottom line: Can you communicate your thoughts effectively? Can you communicate that you're listening or at least send the message back that you're listening to each side of an issue? And are you fair?" Others stressed the value of being able to communicate a mission, vision, and strategy.

Respondents also described business and management or hard skills as important to leadership and command of medical facilities. These leaders described the need for finance, logistics, and general business skills to effectively lead and manage an MTF—for example, understanding budgets, contracts, and metrics; being facile with personnel and other administrative systems; and having a strong foundation in financial and human capital management. Among Navy respondents, several were quick to note, however, that possessing hard skills and knowing how to manage did not equate to leadership.

Many respondents believed that leaders needed "enterprise" knowledge, skills, and abilities.

Across the services, leaders used a variety of terms to describe a need for leaders to possess what we characterize as "enterprise" skills, knowledge, and abilities. Repeatedly in interviews, respondents spoke about the importance of being "systems thinkers," understanding and operationalizing a strategic vision, being a "forward thinker" who proactively addresses issues, and understanding the whole organization and service-specific system, possessing a "global perspective." One Navy leader described such officers as "mature decisionmakers with systems-level thinking ability" who can "think ahead, . . . find the next surprise before it hits you in the face [and can] understand risk and operational or organizational risk management."

Most respondents attested to the value of leaders' understanding of how the other services operate and acknowledged that DoD is increasingly moving toward a more joint system, but they were more mixed in their views about mandatory joint qualifications.

In most interviews, we asked respondents their opinions about the extent to which executive leaders needed joint experience and education and whether they believed that these requirements should be mandatory. Many respondents referred to *joint* as interoperability, integration, and interdependence with other services rather than referencing formal joint billets. One respondent discussed the different conceptions of *joint* directly:

> *Joint* is a word that is thrown around cavalierly and remains not defined. There are some who would say joint means green. There are some [to whom] joint means interoperable, and there are some [to whom] joint means interchangeable.

At a minimum, all respondents seemed to endorse the need for leaders to possess better joint "awareness" and experience. Several noted that because the military has been heading toward joint operations, it is important for officers to gain exposure to and learn about the language, systems, tools, and so on of the other services. Others emphasized that, due to the wars, joint operations are more common. In fact, many leaders gave examples of situations in which joint knowledge and skills would be particularly valuable.

Nevertheless, respondents differed in terms of how far they wanted to endorse requirements regarding joint education and assignments. Some leaders believed that it should be mandatory for high-level leaders (e.g., general, flag) to obtain joint experience and education. Others were more skeptical about mandatory requirements for obtaining joint education and training. Many respondents noted that there are limited joint billets and opportunities to attend JPME. Others were more critical of the content of JPME and its value for leaders. Still others did not believe that all leaders needed joint qualifications. For example, one believed that this knowledge was more valuable to warfighters than to leaders in health care settings. Another saw joint requirements leading to a loss of productivity. Still another felt that training dollars for medical leaders would be better spent on ensuring that they are clinically prepared. (Joint education and training are discussed in more depth later in this chapter.)

There were mixed views on the extent to which military health care leaders should possess and maintain clinical skills.

In general, most respondents believed that leaders needed to have clinical credibility but disagreed about the extent to which credibility required executive leaders to maintain clinical skills and be physicians. Thus, many respondents felt strongly that leaders needed to have excelled in their clinical field and that this expertise helped establish their credibility.

Some respondents took this further, stating that the greatest credibility as a military health care leader comes from being a physician. For example, one Navy leader noted that older generations, in particular, wanted to be led by an MC provider, not a nurse or MSC member: "It's very tough for them to suddenly have a nurse come in when they've been used to doctors running things." Similarly, an Army respondent believed that non-MC providers were at a disadvantage and had a reputation for being "too far distanced from clinical medicine." The Air Force had an explicit policy that medical centers and hospitals (bedded facilities) were to be led by physicians. However, some Air Force leaders felt that this policy was out of step with practice in the civilian world, where hospital leaders are often not physicians. Some respondents in other services also noted that nonphysician leaders were as effective as physician leaders. An Army leader stated, "I think a doctor, a nurse, or an administrator can effectively command a hospital. It's an immaterial job. You've got to know clinical, you've got to have a clinical understanding, you've got to have leadership, but you do have to [be] savvy on business practices." Another set of respondents argued that leaders needed to maintain clinical skills. Thus, a few commanders in all three services described efforts to maintain a certain number of clinical hours and to see patients, stressing the value of doing so. These leaders believed that maintaining at least a limited clinical practice helps one understand what occurs throughout the MTF, thus improving the ability to lead and bolstering credibility. "It also keeps you in touch with the organization," said one Navy leader (a member of the MSC). "If you're never seeing patients, you've . . . lost track of what you're there for in some ways or lost the reality of the day to day."

However, many other respondents disagreed with these assessments of what it means to be clinically competent. Some felt strongly that it was impractical for senior leaders to continue practicing while also fulfilling their many other leadership duties. One Army respondent noted that it is often easier for certain specialties to retain clinical skills, such as a dermatologist compared to a surgeon. This same leader identified other equally valuable ways to maintain clinical competence, such as attending conferences, staying up to date on academic research, and participating in continuing medical education. One Air Force leader noted that credibility did not necessarily require that a leader still operate in the clinics but instead that a leader has "come from that world . . . has been there . . . can empathize and understand that world."

Finally, a few respondents warned against an overemphasis on clinical skills and competence. One Navy leader (MC) cautioned that clinical skills are not sufficient and do not always translate to leadership skills:

> If you just look at somebody strictly for their technical ability and you don't see how they use their technical ability to help expand the entire clinical environment, then maybe they don't have leadership skills.

Some respondents, particularly those in the Army, identified values and character as important attributes of medical leaders.

Several Army respondents described the importance of being honest and open, living by Army values, and having strong character and humility. For example, one Army leader noted,

> The older I get, the things that I value most [are] . . . the values. It's the honesty, it's the integrity, it's the ability to tell the whole truth. Those are extremely important to me. If I have somebody who functions well as a leader, at least the appearance is there, but [if] I can't trust them, then I don't want them to be a leader in my organization.

Although particularly prevalent and explicit in our Army interviews, the topic came up in a few Navy interviews as well and may have been more implicit in some of the other comments. For example, one Navy respondent believed that leaders needed to be fair, demonstrate integrity, and offer to "give 100 percent"; another believed that leaders at this level needed to be highly committed to what they do.

Other respondents referred to educational background and knowledge as important criteria for leaders.

While some cited the value of possessing advanced degrees or completing particular courses, a few respondents also noted that leaders generally needed to demonstrate academic success, knowledge, and intellectual capability.

In all three services, several respondents identified the need for leaders to be flexible and adaptable.

Once again, this theme was particularly strong in the Army interviews, in which many leaders used the words "adaptive," "adapts well," "adaptable," and "agility" when asked to identify what defines an ideal medical leader in the Army. Most believed that it was important for leaders to be able to adapt to changing conditions, particularly those that inevitably result from new positions and frequent moves. We heard similar comments from a few Air Force and Navy respondents.

Although some respondents in all three services were aware of a set of formal leadership competencies endorsed by DoD, most did not remember the name (JMESP), and few found them to be particularly meaningful for measuring or developing leaders.

Across the services, few respondents mentioned these competencies without being solicited to do so. When probed about particular competencies that the military expects from leaders (often a follow-up to another question about how their service defines an ideal leader), many respondents referred to the JMESP competencies—but rarely by name. Although these respondents were aware of a list of 40 competencies (recently reduced to 39, as noted earlier), they often did not remember the name or acronym. More importantly, most of these respondents did not view these competencies as particularly meaningful or consequential. According to one Air Force leader, "[JMESP] is not really utilized . . . in picking or developing [Air Force] leaders." Similarly, a Navy leader explained,

> Would somebody not be selected for a leadership position that hadn't made sure they ticked all the boxes? I don't think that's the case, but, on the other hand, I think most of us . . . felt that it was important that we tried to tick as many of those boxes as we could.

Most respondents also characterized these competencies as something you "get" or "obtain," not demonstrate. One Navy leader noted that there is no standardized method for determining whether people actually gain these competencies. According to other leaders from the Army and Navy, officers submit to the system or "fill in the blocks" that they have "achieved" the necessary competencies through a variety of experiences, but this reporting does not guarantee or even demonstrate that officers have mastered the competencies.

Approach to Leader Development

Although our interview questions emphasized leader development—how and when individuals are identified for leader development opportunities and the specific opportunities provided—respondents often described who is *selected* as a leader and when. This likely had to do with how they and the services define leadership development, much of which depends on experience (i.e., you give someone the opportunity to lead and gain on-the-job experience to develop them as a leader). As a result, the following themes represent both areas: identifying leaders and identifying individuals for leader development. In this section, we outline three components of an approach to leader development—how to select, how to develop, and how to incentivize—but recognize that these categories may overlap. We begin with a few themes regarding the services' overall approach to leader development.

There was variation across and within the services in terms of respondents' perceptions of how purposeful and systematic the services are in developing leaders.

Most Air Force respondents considered the Air Force to have a reasonable and well-defined system in place for leader development. Almost everyone referred to the flight path that provides an overview of the career trajectories for officers by corps. Several respondents also described development teams as the formal process for managing careers.

Perceptions were more mixed in the other two services. Among Army respondents, there was significant disagreement about the extent to which the Army is purposeful and proactive in identifying and developing leaders. At one end of the spectrum, one leader strongly believed that the AMEDD has not done a good job of identifying and grooming high-potentials and relies too heavily on subjective means:

> You have to be willing to mentor and groom anyone, whatever their corps, whatever they look like, and just say, "This is a person I see with leadership potential, and I need to try and expose it and see where this goes." We have not done that in the Army Medical Department. . . . I have watched a couple of those officers [who will speak out] to the right people; next thing you know, they're in command . . . they're going to war college. They haven't had any experience . . . and it's wrong.

Another leader suggested that career progression in the Army is "based on timing and being in the right place at the right time." Another leader added, "Sometimes, we make an effort to grow everybody as that leader versus identifying the 10 or 20 percent to focus on, and that's a challenge as well."

In contrast, other Army leaders perceived a greater sense of purpose in the process of selecting and developing leaders. They described the Army's overall approach as identifying potential leaders and giving them positions of leadership to "see how they do." For example, one leader cited personal experiences over the years that provided "the sense that people have sort of purposely [been] moving me into these positions. 'Let's see how he does with this; let's see how he does with that.'"

Navy respondents also differed greatly in their perceptions of the Navy's approach to leader development. Some characterized the approach as lacking purposeful planning and design, using words such as "happenstance," "luck," and "serendipity" to describe the process of identifying, assigning, and developing leaders. Some reported that development opportunities depended on "what's available at the right time." One leader explained,

> We do not identify our people early enough in their pipeline to get them groomed for training. If it happens, it happens, sort of, . . . by people serendipitously follow[ing] the right track. Or they happen to luck into somebody who kind of grabs them by the shoulders and says, "This is what I want you to start doing at this point in your life." . . . We do it a little better in the Medical Service Corps and in the Nurse Corps, but in the Medical Corps, there's just a lot more haphazard nature to it.

Another Navy respondent characterized development as "haphazard" because (1) individuals who are not qualified to lead are often selected for leader development because other, more qualified candidates are deployed; (2) too much learning is expected to occur on the job; and (3) decisions about who receives development opportunities, such as mentoring and coursework, rely heavily on "serendipity." In contrast, another Navy respondent described a more purposeful process and had already identified a successor.

How to Select
All three services were said to identify high-potential officers, but some respondents reported concerns about this process.

Perhaps reflecting the Air Force's recent work in this area (described in Chapter Three), Air Force respondents were generally positive about their service's systematic process of force development, in which high-potentials are identified and given bigger jobs, commands, and specialized training. As one Air Force leader reported,

> The high-potential ones are given leadership positions very early in rank. . . . Once we identify the ones that we feel have true potential, we push them to bigger jobs,

bigger leadership jobs, even at the intermediate command or the major command level. And we identify them for special training programs. . . . I think the Medical Service Corps is pretty good at identifying the ones that we think have high potential and specifically targeting them for training or job opportunities.

Navy and Army respondents were more mixed in their reports about their services' efforts to identify individuals for leadership and leader development. For example, some Navy respondents believed that the Navy's approach to selection was overly subjective. While one felt that the process relied too heavily on "who you know," another believed that the criteria for selecting leaders varied according to who sat on the selection board. This latter respondent explained that the same individual could be passed up several times by the board and then get selected when the makeup of the selection board changed. As noted earlier, several Navy leaders also argued that rank consciousness often prevented the Navy from identifying true high-potentials.

Finally, across the services, some respondents identified the challenge of identifying the "quiet leaders," acknowledging that in the current system, the more aggressive officers often got the attention. As one Air Force leader explained, "I think the fast burners, the folks that get out there and make the contribution and do their thing, they get identified early." Similarly, several Army respondents noted that it is not always easy to look beyond the more assertive individuals—referred to as "gunners," "go-getters," or "self-selected"—to identify the less vocal ones with potential. One Army MC leader urged for improved efforts to identify these "silent leaders" so as not to miss out on people with the "real, true inner quality of a leader—the motivation skills, communication skills, people skills."

> [There are] a lot of silent leaders out there that would love the opportunity to have some executive skills early on, and then the pool from which you could select your leaders would be much bigger. . . . But we don't offer them the opportunity. We don't go out and be proactive and say, "Is that what you'd like to do?" I think the Nurse Corps does much better than we do, much better.

All services used formal and informal methods to select high-potentials, but perceptions about the efficacy of these methods varied.

Evaluations. Most respondents in all three services described the importance of formal evaluation reports, and many viewed them as one of the primary methods for identifying individuals with leadership potential. For example, according to several Air Force respondents, receiving a below-the-zone promotion and "getting ranked" in one's evaluation are the indicators of high potential. Similarly, several Army respondents noted that officer evaluation reports (OERs) were used to flag individuals to whom the Army should pay attention. In the Air Force, respondents felt that ranking sent a clear signal of who was a high-potential officer and who was not. Ranking was seen as a powerful indicator and a clear message to promotion boards.

Nevertheless, there was widespread concern about the limitations of these reports. First, many leaders commented that evaluations were often inflated. One Navy leader described a "say-do gap" in which the report "may be glowing, but, in reality, the individual may not have a skill set that aligns with what I need." One Air Force respondent stated, "I joke that the worst thing you can ever give someone is an honestly fair evaluation, because without the inflation, they would be at the bottom of the barrel." And although many Army leaders observed improvements resulting from the overhaul of the OER system (using the "above center mass" rule) and acknowledged that the new system prevented "major inflation," they nonetheless believed that the reports were often inflated. "You never comment on a person's negative attributes unless you think that person's going to be a detriment to the corps," said one Army leader. Another Army respondent mentioned inflationary trends and pressures, noting that, especially in war, it is difficult to give officers negative evaluations. Some leaders reported developing strategies over the years to filter information from formal evaluations to identify individuals with true leadership potential, detecting "code words" and "discriminators" in the text.

Other leaders voiced concerns about subjectivity and variable quality of evaluation reports. One Navy leader described the evaluation system as "individualistic," noting that the rater greatly influences the results. This respondent cited the example of an extrovert who was working for an introvert. The introvert thought that efforts to advance interpersonal relations were a waste of time, but the extrovert was actually very successful in developing a network. The converse could also be true, with an introvert working for an extrovert who regards the introvert's attention to detail as nitpicking. Neither would get a high efficiency report because of inherent personality differences, not because of performance.

Similarly, one Army leader complained that senior raters are often too removed or are tasked to rate too many individuals at one time to write meaningful evaluations. Other Army leaders felt strongly that without input from subordinates, OERs provided incomplete information. A few Air Force leaders also believed that evaluations could be problematic if a rater does not possess good writing skills and that "careers can be ruined" because of this failure.

Selection and Command Boards. Many respondents also mentioned the role that boards play in identifying and selecting individuals for leadership and leader development, yet they varied in their perceptions of the "soundness" of this process. Some were fairly positive. For example, one Army leader believed that the board process was extremely sound, and, while OERs were inflated, "the officers who sit on those boards . . . know that and [are] looking for other discriminators within that record."

As mentioned earlier, others voiced concerns about the boards' subjectivity. For example, one Navy leader believed that the criteria for selecting leaders depended significantly on who sat on the selection board. This respondent explained that the same individual could be passed over several times by the board and then be selected when the makeup of the selection board changed. Similarly, an Army leader commented, "You can have a perfectly developed and executed leader development program, but when you're relying on a centralized board process to then select those officers and place them into commands—leadership positions—the outcome is strongly influenced by the board composition."

Interviews. A few leaders mentioned interviews as another formal and effective way to select leaders. Two Army leaders stressed that interviews provide information that OERs and other written documents cannot, such as details about individual motivations. Two Navy leaders indicated that interviewing may be increasing throughout the Navy. One felt that any admiral who was serious about what he or she was doing would use personal interviews to fill positions and not rely entirely on detailers' advice. Another individual who had been interviewed along with 12 others (mentioning that this was something the Navy had started doing recently) thought that it was a useful process and another way to identify high performers.

One Air Force respondent described interviews as being used to fill some positions but not those at the highest levels of command.

Reputation and Word of Mouth. Many leaders across the services noted that an "informal system" of information gleaned from colleagues and word of mouth greatly affected the identification of leaders. Several Army leaders mentioned relying on key leaders to recognize "rising stars" and learning about high-potential officers from colleagues who called or sent email messages (e.g., "You really need to look after Captain Smith because he is one who we need to groom to be a future leader ten to 15 years from now"). Some argued that these informal networks were often more important than formal methods of selecting leaders at the highest levels. One Air Force leader stated that when the senior leadership got together, they looked for recommendations from others:

> When we're looking at folks to fill the senior-level positions and, say, especially on the staffs—not the squadron commanders, or not the group commanders, but the staff—you say, "Hey, this'll be a great guy, did a great job for us over here at Pacific Air Forces. I think he'd do a great job on the Air Staff." So there's a lot of exchange of information that goes on, yes, at the senior level.

A Navy respondent echoed this belief: "As they move up into the more . . . senior executive roles, fitness reports . . . in my personal opinion play less of a role [than] service reputation and word of mouth."

A few Navy respondents raised concerns about attention to diversity in the selection of leaders and potential leaders.

Perhaps due to the fact that the Navy has been formally working on this issue, several Navy leaders explicitly mentioned diversity when describing selection procedures. One leader observed that the military had not made an adequate commitment to ensuring diversity of not only gender and race but also "diversity of mind" and viewpoints among its leaders:

> I think that's the one challenge that people have in leadership is do you want to grow an organization that looks like you, or do you truly want a diverse, dynamic organization that can adapt and move into the future?

Similarly, another leader commented on the homogeneity of leadership and believed that although some attention was being paid to diversity, not enough was being done to change patterns: "If we keep on bringing in the same people who are going through the same process, we're going to end up with the same outcome, the same product."

Respondents expressed a range of opinions about the timing of identification for leadership and leader development opportunities.

Many respondents across the services felt strongly that identification needed to occur early in one's career. One Air Force respondent thought that potential leaders should be identified as early as possible, developed, and treated according to their potential, stating,

> I think we need to try to identify them early, . . . but . . . we need to realize that we have some special people, and we need to treat them specially.

Several leaders in the Army and Navy argued that identification needed to occur earlier than it currently does. For example, many Navy leaders believed that formal development opportunities often come too late in one's career to be useful. One leader was adamant that the Navy needed to be more proactive in providing opportunities to individuals before they are in a leadership position, rather than offering them "after the fact."

This leader went on to explain how various financial, legal, and management courses would have been valuable if taken prior to promotion to a leadership position because they could have provided a better framework to answer pertinent leadership questions: "What do I need to ask about? What are higher-level people looking at?" Another respondent was critical of an assumption that individuals can learn business skills on the job and believed that formal training was necessary before taking on a leadership position: "You can't afford to learn that for the first time when you take over one of these organizations." Finally, several other Navy respondents acknowledged that, often, the "timing doesn't work out" because certain courses are oversubscribed, not enough slots are available, or individuals are forced to take on a new position quickly. As a result, individuals cannot get into the course until after they have taken on the new position for which the course is intended to prepare them.

In all three services, leaders mentioned that doctors do not receive leader development opportunities early enough in their careers. For example, one Army physician leader felt strongly that some leadership development could occur as early as one's residency program, saying, "We have to begin intentionally training our CEOs when they're captains and majors. I think it's true in [the] civilian [world] as well."

Nevertheless, a few outliers did not think that leader development and selection should occur earlier. Some respondents were satisfied with the current timing of selection. One Army leader felt that the Army identified individuals when they were too young and cut off opportunities for some who had potential. A few Navy leaders discussed the challenge of determining the right timing for training. One respondent suggested that if it were offered too early in a career, the individual would have no experience to which he or she could apply the new knowledge: "Back when they did send me to the formal school, there was a lot of it that was not that important to me at the time." However, others indicated that if development and selection were delayed too long, the information and learning might no longer be useful and simply repeat what is already known or learned from experience.

How to Develop

Job Assignments. Respondents highlighted the value of diverse job assignments, as well as on-the-job experiences, for leader development.

Across all three services, almost all respondents described job assignments as a key method for developing leaders.

Some respondents were explicit about the ways in which job experience built specific skills, such as learning how a budget works, how to hire and fire individuals, and so on. Others noted that on-the-job experience allows leaders to interact with individuals across the organization and across corps, which enhances their knowledge about others' responsibilities and their ability to communicate and lead. ("If you're going to be effective, get out there and talk to them.")

Many leaders viewed on-the-job experience as the most valuable and effective means of developing leaders. For example, one Army leader commented, "[Formal] courses lay a very marginal foundation for success. . . . Nothing takes the place of [experience in] getting you ready for becoming a leader down the road." Similarly, an Air Force respondent said, "The best way to learn anything is by doing it. . . . By doing it, I've learned so much more than I would ever have learned in any textbook or course or discussions." A Navy leader also noted that because leadership is so difficult to teach or train, development occurs most effectively when people are given opportunities to lead and then are provided with feedback and mentoring.

Not all respondents were satisfied with the emphasis on developing leaders through job assignments, however. Some Navy respondents characterized the Navy's approach to leader development as development "by fire," in which individuals are thrown into leadership positions and unfairly expected to acquire the necessary skills on the job. For example, when asked whether the Navy has programs to give technically skilled individuals (e.g., doctors) training before they assume executive positions, one leader responded, "They're just thrown in there and the assumption is that you're going to try to acquire it." Another respondent concurred that this is a particular challenge for the MC, in which great physicians were suddenly thrust into XO positions and required to be "a comptroller, [know] materiel management, facilities, base ops, [be] a business manager, a mentor, a coach, disciplinarian, . . . and a judge." In other words, such officers undergo trial by fire and do well because they are exceptional people, but they do not receive formal training.

Similarly, an Army leader believed that the Army could do a better job of giving leadership experience to potential leaders so that they are not exposed to the demands of the job for the first time when they are put in charge of an organization:

> Offer them pieces of those positions or [give] them an opportunity to sit in those positions for periods of time to have that exposure, so that when they're there the first time it isn't when they're in charge.

Many respondents argued that diversity of job experience is important for leader development.

For instance, one leader described the need to be a "well-rounded leader," which included a diversity of experience and "wide exposure" to different types of jobs and responsibilities. Related to this, respondents from each of the services described a system by which individuals are given opportunities to experience increasing levels of responsibility and scopes of work, each role expanding their skills and knowledge as a leader. One Air Force leader explained how the progression of job experience builds different skills and increasingly broad views of the system that future generals need. For example, as an officer progresses from being a doctor to a flight surgeon to a squadron commander,

> you're no longer just thinking about your flight surgeon's office. You're thinking about aerospace medicine, . . . about public health, . . . about biomedical engineering, . . . about health promotions.

In addition, the respondent noted that a good squadron commander needed to learn what other squadrons were doing, to learn to compromise and work with others.

Ultimately, as the officer progressed further up the chain, he or she would begin to understand the missions of many different bases. The respondent concluded,

> So I think it's experience, it's exposure. I think you need to move and you have to [experience] leadership at all different levels.

Several individuals identified not only jobs but also certain job experiences that equated to leader development opportunities.

For example, one Army respondent regularly urged other leaders to "prepare their bench" by allowing high-potentials to represent them at meetings or by putting them in charge when the leaders were on leave. That respondent explained, citing personal experience, "That's the way you learn." Others described ways for individuals to take on leadership development "roles" and "duties." For instance, one Army official explained that there are many opportunities for physicians to step up and take on leadership roles, such as being service chief, being department chief, being in charge of a joint commission, and serving on committees. The respondent noted that leaders needed "to step forward and take on these leadership roles, and those are the growing jobs." Two respondents mentioned collateral duties as another means of developing leaders. These duties, such as serving on or chairing a committee, were viewed as useful ways to provide clinical staff leadership experience and experience with "the administrative side of things" while still allowing officers to remain in their clinical positions.

Another Army leader provided several examples of intentionally being given opportunities to lead by serving on committees and described how these opportunities fostered the development of new knowledge and skills:

> [A leader] directed a zero-based budget review of the entire hospital budget . . . [and] I was the physician representative. . . . The best thing was the exercise for me, because I know what zero-based budgeting is now. . . . And then the same thing— he decided he wanted someone to chair the performance-improvement council that had traditionally been chaired by the general, and somehow it ended up being me.

Similarly, an Air Force leader described helping potential leaders experience greater command levels on a temporary basis:

> As I'm selecting people within my group or within my wing for leadership positions, I will very deliberately pull people out and put them in temporary positions, at least, where I know they're out of their element, because I want to push them. I want to see how they can expand into that mission environment.

A few respondents described other on-the-job experiences, such as fellowships, internships, and staff positions, as methods of developing leaders.

Air Force respondents described several programs:

You can do a readiness fellowship, for instance, at the air combat command. . . . There's several fellowships out there, and we're always trying to identify those opportunities where we could offer fellowships to basically develop future leaders.

One program . . . that has been very beneficial to identify high-performing leaders early is the Air Force intern program, and that is a way of identifying captains and getting them into various positions at the Pentagon or the Air Staff to expose them early in their career to some of the senior leadership decisions, strategic and operational planning, and that is a very good foundation for our more junior-grade officers.

Similarly, a Navy leader noted that certain staff positions allow people to gain more experience and exposure. For example, this leader took on a policy-level position at one point, which provided a "very good overview of the bigger enterprise and what executive medicine would be like." The leader noted that others take on detailer positions or positions in Health Affairs to determine whether they are interested in leadership.

Across the services, many leaders considered joint experience to be beneficial to leader development; however, only a few leaders thought that such experience should be mandatory.

Some respondents strongly endorsed the need for joint assignments. As noted earlier, some respondents cited the value of operating with other services and learning to "speak a joint language." One Army leader argued for an expanded definition of "joint" and for opportunities to develop joint skills and knowledge through assignments (for example, with agencies and tours with coalition partners). This respondent thought joint assignments should occur early but also believed that an officer who demonstrated potential but had reached the rank of colonel without a joint assignment could still get joint experience as a colonel. The respondent further argued that joint experience was important enough to formalize the requirement in AMEDD.

While many leaders saw benefits in joint experience, few respondents thought that it should be mandatory, due to a lack of billets. Even an Air Force leader who described joint experience as "essential" noted that it could not be made mandatory because there are so few slots for medical leaders. As a Navy leader put it, "My gut feeling says . . . because there are so few jobs . . . you would lose some quality people."

Interestingly, a couple of Army leaders were concerned about the consequences of moving more medical leaders into joint assignments. One believed that it would lead to a loss of productivity. Another thought that it would interfere with the mission of providing warrior care. Yet another noted that AMEDD would need to grow in size to offset the loss of positions.

One Air Force leader argued that what was needed was for a certain number of the highest-level leaders to have joint experience:

> It's not necessary that all our general officers have joint experience. . . . But I think you need a certain number . . . in the joint job, because you need to have that perspective also at the senior leadership position.

Education and Training. Respondents had mixed views on the education and training opportunities offered by the services. They valued the opportunities provided by external organizations but also recognized barriers to participating in such programs.

Respondents described a number of educational opportunities provided to officers as they moved up the career ladder.

Almost everyone described formal education and training received for certain positions and commands. Army respondents mentioned the Command and General Staff College and other executive leader courses. Similarly, Navy leaders spoke about XO and CO courses and tracks, as well as the capstone course. One Air Force leader described the progression of education and training for MSC officers:

> We start off with a three-month course . . . called Health Services Administration for all new MSC officers. . . . Then, we develop some people with internships in certain fields, like logistics. We start them off with an internship for about ten months, then they go off and take a staff position someplace in a hospital or clinic. . . . Then, . . . we also have fellowships that we offer, usually at the senior captain or major level, where they . . . work with a major command. . . . In some cases, they are also at an area hospital level. We have a fellowship, for example, in medical readiness. . . . We also do education with industry. And we send people off for master's degrees, too, usually at the lieutenant and junior captain level. And, of course, the PME . . . is factored in for Medical Service Corps officers.

A couple of Navy respondents described training and education that focused on the larger goals of the Navy rather than their specific positions. For example, one noted a strong emphasis on human capital management in recent years. Another described the progression over the years from a focus on management to Total Quality Management to Lean Six Sigma. That respondent explained it as "the black belt, and green belt, and blue belt, whatever it is. So sort of as you grow, you do whatever the interest is of your service."

In general, there were mixed views about the value of the current education and training offered by the services.

Some respondents were proponents of various offerings and believed that certain courses were valuable. Others were more middle-of-the-road, noting that courses and training provide exposure to important information, but true learning comes from on-the-job experiences (as discussed earlier). As one Army leader noted, formal centralized educational provides some useful training on "how to command" and some exposure to budget and finance issues but that, "really, you've got to get out there and do that to learn all that stuff." Several leaders noted the need for additional content in educational opportunities provided by the services. Leaders across the services cited a need for more instruction on the business aspects of medicine, such as finance and budgeting (particularly for clinicians), as well as writing skills.

All respondents described senior-level PME opportunities offered to leaders, including their service's war college and the National War College, yet they held mixed views of their value.

Attending the National War College in residence was described as prestigious and a marker for flag officer potential. As one Air Force respondent noted, "Officers who go to those courses are destined [for] higher levels of responsibility." Leaders across the services noted the limited number of in-residence slots at the National War College. However, respondents within and across the services differed in their opinions about the value of these opportunities and whether in-residence opportunities should be expanded for medical leaders.

In the Air Force, respondents considered attending senior PME courses in residence to be far more beneficial than completing them by means of correspondence. War college by correspondence was considered something that "checked a box." A couple of respondents who completed through correspondence found the content to be too focused on the line: "It's geopolitics, and it's joint warfare, and it's warfighting thinking . . . and it's not, 'Can you run a hospital?'" However, another leader disagreed with that rationale, noting that medical leaders needed to develop as military officers, not just as medical officers:

> I think that the way the Air Force approaches PME . . . [is] the right approach. . . .
> I have heard people in the medical field say that they think it's too line-centric. . . .
> Air Force PME gives a good, broad picture of what we should be learning about.
> It's really a course to learn about how to be a military officer more than it is how
> to be a medical professional, a communications professional, a pilot. . . . It's above
> career fields, and it's more . . . what an officer needs to be educated on. . . . I think
> medical officers do need to understand the entire Air Force picture, and PME is
> one of the best ways to get that.

In fact, the majority of Air Force respondents found these PME opportunities very valuable, particularly those who attended in residence. However, when asked whether medical leaders should receive additional slots to allow more to attend in residence, almost no Air Force leaders agreed with such a policy. As one officer noted, "Oh, it would be beneficial to the medics, but it would be detrimental to the line because you only have two other spots, so I would leave it like it is."

In the Army, some leaders valued the senior service colleges and the U.S. Army War College, but several noted barriers to participation. One leader described the senior service colleges as the single best preparation for a command position. Others noted that they learned a lot from attending the Army War College (e.g., strategic thinking, "how to think outside just the Army box") and believed that more seats were needed. However, several strongly favored the residence option over the distance program but recognized the difficulty of selecting that option. One leader noted that the online program does not offer the valuable opportunity to network and interact with other officers. Another described the distance learning program as "painful." Several acknowledged that participating in the residence option was difficult if one has a family. For example, one leader chose to forgo the opportunity to avoid disrupting their child's education.

Several Army leaders expressed a need for new joint education opportunities. For example, one respondent believed that joint education could be integrated into the captain's career course and other intermediate-level education (ILE). The respondent argued that JPME could be distilled to a three- to four-month joint course for medical professionals. Another simply noted that "the curriculum of the course can't be so onerous that the doctors won't sign up."

In the Navy, several respondents criticized the war colleges and senior service colleges, particularly for the amount of time it took to complete courses. One leader said that it is especially difficult for doctors to drop what they are doing and that the time required results in the loss of their bonus. Many were also concerned about the limited number of spots available in these programs. Several believed that the military needed to come up with another option, for example, training that is tailored to medical leaders to familiarize them with how the other services work, or infusing some of this education into existing, standard courses. Another felt strongly that all programs should be conducted online. Finally, one respondent argued that those who are selected for war college did not always apply what they learned to their subsequent positions because the Navy was not thoughtful in how it assigned individuals after they attended these programs, noting that some schools' seats were filled based on who was available to take the courses offered. Furthermore, follow-on assignments after graduation did not necessarily take advantage of the material learned in the course, and, often, a pressing need to fill a billet took precedence over utilizing knowledge and skills learned in the advanced school.

Respondents across the services identified the value of educational and training opportunities provided by individuals and organizations outside of the military.

In many cases, these outside opportunities were sponsored by the services, such as graduate school attendance. One Army leader recalled a valuable strategic leadership course offered by the Army that brought in industry leaders:

> I learned so much. And he brought in CEOs from other companies and we had a chance to interact with them to tell them how we do business, and we were able to learn about how they execute as CEOs. I thought that was very effective in terms of looking outside the military.

Several respondents described the Interagency Institute for Federal Health Care Executives at George Washington University. All respondents who attended this program found it beneficial because it focused on health care and provided an opportunity for interagency perspectives. One Air Force respondent said,

> So, it gives you an opportunity to understand that there are other folks out there, potentially they could be your allies, or potentially vying for the same resources. . . . In order for us to win this global war on terrorism, I would argue that the DoD is probably 15 percent of the solution. The other 85 percent of that is the interagency. . . . And I understood that a little bit better before [my next assignment in a joint command] because of, again, having the exposure to some of these other [agencies] through the National War College.

In other cases, leaders across the services described seeking education outside the military. One Navy leader believed that at the senior executive level, most individuals sought courses outside the military because the military did not provide equivalent opportunities. This leader was particularly appreciative of ACHE courses.

However, a few respondents reported that lack of time is a barrier to participating in formal education and training.

As one Navy leader explained, "At the senior level, many don't have the time" to enroll in educational offerings like a master's program. As a result, the respondent believed that these master's programs would never be a "major pathway" for development or a "major tool in my quiver." Another noted that the time commitment to attend war college was a problem.

While such courses can be a method of improving access to educational opportunities for busy leaders, respondents expressed mixed views about the value of online education. For instance, several leaders across the services believed that enrolling in war college online removed the valuable experience of interacting and networking with other officers. However, others—particularly in the Navy—noted some benefits to online courses. One leader stated that online courses aided in self-education because some people felt freer to speak up and share their opinions in that venue. Another respondent thought that more distance education options were needed for the

Captains Career Course because, without this option, not enough physicians had the opportunity to take the course.

Mentoring. Respondents agreed that mentoring was important for leader development and believed that informal mentoring arrangements were more effective than formal programs.

There was widespread agreement across services that mentoring was important for leader development, and almost all respondents described personal experiences of mentoring or being mentored.

Mentor relationships were initiated from both the top and the bottom. Respondents across the services described reaching out to a specific senior officer based on common interests. As one Army leader put it, "I just chose my own mentors . . . because I wanted to be more like them and I saw them do things that I valued." Other respondents talked about looking for young officers to mentor and the desire to "find your replacement." Many described the importance of "mentoring the next generation of leaders." One Air Force leader explained,

> Each of us in more senior positions, I think, has a 3×5 card where we've written down . . . the dozen or so folks that we have under our wing. . . . That's my favorite part of the job, quite frankly: the young physicians and enlisted members of the team—physicians, nonphysicians, and enlisted members of the team—that come to me for advice.

Another Air Force respondent reiterated the importance of mentoring throughout the life cycle of an officer's career:

> It's very important to capture opportunities and continue to . . . develop our individuals who have that thirst, for growth especially, and then also to seek professional development mentoring from those senior [officers]. . . . I'm just very pleased to be able to share what I have learned and mentor some of the more junior officers developing today.

A few respondents noted that they often served as mentors but never explicitly labeled the relationships in this way. For example, one Army leader noted,

> I've mentored one specific officer from afar for the last several years. . . . I have identified her as a great junior officer and want to make sure that she is challenged and motivated in the right way because she's got so much potential.

A Navy leader spoke of personal experience with informal mentoring:

> I have at least two or three people that have . . . mentored me. And each time, they provide you some of that feedback and the guidance on what jobs to take or what collaterals to take or what areas you need to work on.

An Air Force leader said that mentors help junior leaders understand "where you are, where you need to go, and how to get the needed knowledge set."

While some leaders noted that their service had a formal mentoring system, almost all described informal mentoring and tended to believe that it was more effective than formal mentoring programs.

One Air Force leader described the formal system as a failure that was no longer followed. "We tried a formal mentoring program. . . . And it was just a flop because it was way too formal." Similarly, one Navy leader explained, "We formally talk about it. It informally happens. And again, typically how that happens is kind of [through] individual initiative."

Other respondents felt strongly that mentoring was not successful when it occurred formally. "When it becomes formal," said one leader, "often those who don't really want to be doing it—whether as a mentor or mentee—aren't fully participatory. And so the results aren't as productive as people would like." Similarly, as a Navy leader explained, a mentor relationship cannot be an "assigned thing" because sometimes the two parties do not "click":

> I may look across several directorates or at several other people in jobs above me and say, "This person is someone who I feel comfortable working with," and I'll approach them, talk to them, or they may contact me and say, "Hey, I notice we've got similar interests. Your career path that you look like you're going down is similar to mine." And you establish a relationship in that way. But to dictate it and say, "This [person] is going to be your mentor"—that sounds very military, but that's not really the way we do it.

One Air Force respondent couched this in terms of a "natural" mentorship rather than a formal one.

Only one respondent, however, felt that formal mentoring was preferable to informal mentoring. This leader believed that formal mentoring ensured less sporadic interactions and provided for greater communication. Nevertheless, like the others interviewed, this individual believed that it was critical for the person being mentored to opt into the relationship.

Career Counseling. Respondents described variations in the way the services approached career counseling.

While respondents in each of the services were more likely to value the informal career advice received from mentors over formal career counseling, there were differences among the services in terms of how leaders described the formal career counseling process.

In the Air Force, respondents described career counseling as a part of the formal development team process. One respondent explained that within the past few years, a procedure was implemented wherein the most senior physician from the major commands would review lists of officers selected for promotion to major, lieutenant colonel, and colonel to ascertain career strengths and weaknesses and identify likely assignments for them. Each officer was provided with feedback from this analysis of his or her career and offered a selection of assignments consistent with that career to date. Another Air Force respondent said that people are emailed advice periodically (e.g., "Time for you to consider x") by their development team.

However, in the Navy, few respondents discussed career counseling as a formal leader development strategy. Only one respondent mentioned the midterm counseling that occurs with the Career Development Board, in which officers talk with more senior officers about career goals and review the steps necessary to reach them.

In the Army, some respondents cited the value of having received career counseling in their own careers, although they often noted that it was something they sought out on their own (self-selected development rather than systematic). One leader recalled being a captain and sitting down with a supervisor to develop a career map, returning to it many times over the years. This same respondent acknowledged seeking out counseling and career advice from the various leaders for whom the respondent had worked over the years. Another leader similarly recalled sitting down as a lieutenant with a mentor and preparing a 20-year plan in five-year increments.

Further, some Army leaders identified a need for more career counseling early in one's career. One respondent acknowledged having "no idea these positions exist[ed]" in early career phases and that it would be valuable to communicate and prepare officers early to think about their future. Similarly, another leader believed that officers needed assistance early in their careers to assess where they want to be in the future and whether they want to be commanders.

Feedback. When it was mentioned, 360-degree feedback was seen as an important component of leader development.

In the Army and Navy, a few respondents mentioned the 360-degree evaluation process and feedback as a way of fostering leader development.

One Army leader explained that, as part of one ILE leader development cell, officers were encouraged to seek input from those with whom they had recently worked or for whom they had worked a long time ago. The respondent believed that, over time, these anonymous assessments helped reinforce individuals' perceptions of themselves and where they believed their strengths and weaknesses might be. Another leader mentioned the optional 360-degree online process offered through the U.S. Army War College. This particular leader participated in the process and received a 110-page document with input from superiors, subordinates, and peers—input characterized as "a real, pure look" that was not inflated. The respondent described it as "one of the most useful documents I've had in leadership, because it included subordinates and peers and it was very helpful feedback. . . . I learned a lot about myself." The course instructor also spent about two hours reviewing the document with the respondent, which was also valuable.

In the Navy, a commander had participated in a 360-degree process as part of an ACHE course and noted how valuable this feedback was:

> [It] gave you feedback on your own leadership style, your management style, how others perceived you. . . . Not only did you learn about all the different leadership styles and team building and ways to move an organization forward, but you then had some concrete feedback . . . that showed, really, a little bit more about yourself.

While 360-degree evaluations were not mentioned by any of our Air Force respondents, they did describe feedback received through the development team process (see the section "Career Counseling," earlier in this chapter).

Self-Development. Respondents stated that self-initiated development, such as participation in a program or pursuit of a degree, was a feature of their development as leaders.

Respondents in each of the services described self-initiated development as important for leaders.

When describing their own career paths, some leaders characterized their decision to seek out a particular development opportunity (e.g., obtaining a master's degree, attending a particular course) as self-initiated and not something that was recommended or required. Other respondents described taking courses to improve their skills (e.g., budget management, writing), attending conferences organized by civilian organizations, and maintaining certification through civilian accrediting bodies. One Army leader described various "self-help" options for development, such as online courses and reading programs (e.g., Army Surgeon General and corps commander reading programs, division commander and brigade commander recommended reading lists), stating that they provide good foundations and research on various topics (e.g., strategic thinking). The respondent commented, "Everything else is really self-development and self-tracked. So, it depends really on how motivated you are to develop your craft. No one's going to look over you and say, 'Did you read that?'"

In fact, several leaders emphasized that individuals in the military had to take responsibility for seeking out opportunities to improve areas of weakness. According to one Navy leader,

> If you feel like you're struggling . . . in one particular area—let's say budgeting or personnel, . . . it's incumbent upon the person in that position to seek out help, and it's available. . . . It will be recognized eventually that you've got shortfalls in that area, and if you don't do something about it before it comes to the attention of [higher] executives, then you're really going to be setting yourself up for failure.

How to Incentivize

Several respondents across the services described how leaders were incentivized to participate in certain "development opportunities" that were said to greatly affect promotion and command opportunities.

A key example of this was advanced PME courses. Several respondents noted that the only reason some people go through their service's war college or the National War College, particularly by correspondence, is that it is a requirement for promotion. As one Air Force leader explained, "They'll do it just because they want to make colonel, and those who don't do it really don't get promoted."

Similarly, a Navy leader noted that war college attendance was "practically a prerequisite . . . a discriminator when you go through those boards. . . . I recognize that the skills I learned would be necessary to do that job, but I also recognize that it's a discriminator for the board, so that's why I signed up."

Other leaders related their own decision to seek education and assignments to promotion incentives. For example, one Navy commander, a practitioner, sought out the development opportunities that enhanced administrative skills in an effort to become more competitive and get promoted. In other words, the leader was "getting that check in the box." This leader similarly identified promotion as the rationale for attending Naval War College and obtaining an advanced degree:

> Nobody told me I had to take it or it was a requirement, but I knew that it would benefit my career and promotion opportunities if I had taken those classes.

The leader further noted that, although it was not formally documented anywhere, to be promoted to O-6, one needed to complete the courses, and it was understood that these would make the leader more competitive.

Several other leaders noted that the Surgeon General of Navy Medicine declared that he would not select anyone to be an MTF commander unless they had operational experience and, as a result, "a flurry of people that hadn't had it . . . ran over to do it."

A few leaders mentioned that nurses must maintain clinical practice and competence to retain their credentials.

This credentialing requirement served as an incentive for individuals to perform a certain number of clinical hours each year or to attend certain courses that fulfilled this requirement (e.g., advanced cardiac life support).

Many respondents were concerned about whether OERs provided objective feedback.

As noted earlier, many respondents were concerned about the objectivity and fairness of the OERs. For example, insufficient training in how to write such evaluations could disadvantage an individual in the promotion process. Often, senior raters were too far removed from the officer to really know his or her strengths and weaknesses, and, they said, because most OERs were inflated, they did not provide a good assessment of the individual.

Outcome

Across the three services, the vast majority of respondents held very positive views about the skills and abilities of current medical leaders, but many described areas in which leadership skills could be enhanced.

When asked whether there were any areas in which current leaders were not adequately prepared, many cited a lack of business and management skills. Others offered this observation unsolicited when discussing leadership more generally. For example, a few leaders in each of the services believed that clinical leaders needed a better understanding of the administrative side of the house (and the converse as well—that administrators needed a better appreciation of the clinical side of the house). As one Navy leader noted,

> The clinical side often is completely clueless as to anything dealing with administration. For example, dealing with credentials, and privileging, and quality counsel, and quality issues, the hospital administrator frequently doesn't understand. . . . On the clinical side, they seem to have really no idea about IT systems, and why can't we do this, and the budgeting, and the difference between appropriations, what's the difference between operation and maintenance, and other procurement, and things that administration kind of takes for granted. . . . We need to put more emphasis on teaching the clinical side about how administration works, and we need to put more emphasis on the administrators, teaching them how the clinical side works.

Similarly, an Army leader (MSC) commented,

We in the AMEDD . . . have to do a better job of developing all officers to be commanders. . . . You can take a surgeon and put him in as a commander and [he] won't have the same skill sets. They're focused on patient care, where you have to be more open to your entire organization. . . . We have a precommand course in the AMEDD, but it doesn't get to how you deal with your sergeant major, . . . teaching them to be partners—because, out here, you've got to deal with the congressmen. . . . [Doctors are] doing other things throughout their career, and then . . . they come out on the command list. So, I think we have to do a better job [preparing them]. The Medical Service Corps officers—no problems. . . . A few docs . . . are exceptions because they go out and they become division surgeons. But [for] those who stay within the AMEDD, . . . we need to set them up for success.

Some Air Force respondents expressed concerns about how the "best-in-breed" competition affected outcomes. Several individuals thought that the competition within corps resulted in suboptimal leadership choices. As one individual described it, "The best people in the corps may not be the best people for the job."

Other Comments on Improving Leader Development

We asked respondents whether they had advice or thoughts on how to improve leader development in the services. We summarize their responses here.

Many respondents argued that the services needed to identify and provide development opportunities earlier in an officer's career.

As one leader stated, "We have to identify candidates early. It behooves us to identify them early, make them understand early we think they have potential, so they don't get out." This would also increase the military's return on investment. Another respondent believed that junior officers needed strong mentorship early in their careers and that feedback should be offered and counseling should occur regularly and before officers are evaluated. In all three services, respondents mentioned the need to provide physicians with leader development and command opportunities earlier in their careers.

From a Medical Corps perspective, I think what needs to be done is they need to give doctors the opportunity to participate. From the early part of my career, you never really had the opportunity to pull your nose off the patient-care grindstone and indulge an interest in medical or health care management. . . . I think we need to focus a little more on [the period] after the doctor has done his residency and first three to four years of payback time [when he has] solidified his clinical skill sets, affording him the time to attend a four- or six-year-long course, like an MHA [master of health administration] or whatever. I think that would do a lot to foster Medical Corps leaders.

A few leaders offered suggestions for improving the selection process, such as improving OERs and deliberately looking beyond rank.

As noted earlier, several respondents suggested integrating an element of 360-degree evaluations into the official OER process by allowing for peer and subordinate input. Others simply argued for further training and time invested in writing evaluations to make these documents more meaningful. Navy respondents, in particular, urged that service to look beyond rank and give greater emphasis to diversity when selecting officers for leader development.

Several leaders suggested ways to enhance leader development via shorter-term job assignments and experiences.

Suggestions included the creation of a "leader intern" position that would allow people to "try it on for size" before taking time out of their clinical lives to get an advanced degree, participation in committees and commissions that were outside the immediate area of expertise, and fellowships and traineeships. Officers could be encouraged to participate through recognition on their evaluation reports.

Many leaders offered advice on how to improve education and training for leaders.

Several respondents believed that clinical leaders needed more instruction on "the business aspects of medicine," such as budgets, contracts, and pay systems, as well as how to command. Others argued for increased opportunities for JPME (perhaps attached to a degree) and possible opportunities to integrate joint medical training, awareness, and cross-service training into existing courses.

Several respondents mentioned the need to attend to retention issues, especially work-life balance issues and length of assignments.

Increasing the length of the typical assignment to three years would help with both retention and depth of experience in the military.

Several respondents (including some Air Force officers) recommended that the Air Force move away from competition within corps and move back to competition across corps.

One Air Force respondent argued,

I think we need to get away from this kind of careerist, "We need to push *x* number of whatever through the system so they have a promotion opportunity." . . . And I think that's a mistake. . . . We don't need to set a quota.

Others suggested more middle-of-the-road approaches: making job assignments by corps "guidance" rather than a mandate or quota, or providing the option to give command positions to other corps.

Summary of Findings from Interviews

Table 4.1 summarizes the views of the military leaders in our sample with respect to the main categories of leader development.

Table 4.1
Overview of Themes Identified in Interviews with Military Leaders

Area	Findings

Context and organizational environment	Military environment is increasingly complex
	    Need to deal with diverse workforces (military, civilian, contract)
	    Increased turnover due to demands of ongoing wars
	    New productivity requirements

	Differences among corps in opportunities for leadership and growth
	Differences in services' approaches to leader selection: "best in breed" compared with "best in show"
Organizational leader expectations	Experience in a broad set of assignments seen as a critical criterion for leaders Both "hard" and "soft" skills necessary for leaders

	"Enterprise" knowledge/skills/ability mentioned by many as important
	    Consensus that leaders need to know how other services operate
	    Mixed views regarding mandatory joint qualifications for health professions officers

	Mixed views regarding need for leaders to possess and maintain clinical skills
	Values and character, as well as advanced educational degrees, explicitly mentioned by some as important leader attributes
	Flexibility and adaptability also important
	JMESP competencies not explicitly mentioned by name and not seen as particularly meaningful for leader development

Approach to leader development	Varied views about how systematic the services are in developing leaders
	    Current Air Force system seen as reasonable and well defined
	    Perceptions more mixed in Army and Navy—seen as purposeful by some, more "happenstance" by others

Table 4.1—Continued

Area	Findings
How to select: Evaluations Boards Interviews Reputation	Services formally and informally identify high-potential officers, but concerns exist about the process (overly subjective, challenge of identifying "quiet" leaders) and about its effectiveness
	Evaluations and promotion/command boards crucial in selection, but both have limitations (inflation, subjectivity, variable quality, distance between rater and officer)
	Interviews used infrequently but seen as providing information missing from other sources
	Selection strongly influenced by reputation and word of mouth
	Need for leaders to be identified and provided with development opportunities earlier in career mentioned by most Inadequate early leader development opportunities for physicians mentioned by respondents in all three services
How to develop: Job assignments Education and training Mentoring Career counseling Feedback Self-development	Job assignments widely seen as key to development
	Both diversity of experiences and certain key job experiences seen as important
	On-the-job experiences (staff jobs, fellowships) also mentioned by a few as important
	Joint experience seen as beneficial, but few thought it should be mandatory
	Views about value of some formal military education courses mixed
	Educational opportunities outside the military seen as valuable by many
	Lack of time as a barrier to participation in formal education/training mentioned by a few
	Mentoring widely seen as important, but majority found informal mentoring more effective than formal mentoring
	Career counseling part of new formal development process in Air Force; less so in Army (some sought it on their own) and Navy
	360-degree feedback not widely practiced but mentioned by a few as a good leader development approach
	Self-initiated development seen as important
How to incentivize: Promotion or command opportunities Officer evaluations	Education and development opportunities seen as necessary for promotion/command, so eagerly sought-after
	Officer evaluations considered inflated and may not provide good feedback
Outcome	Positive perceptions of skills and abilities of current leaders, but areas for improvement identified Business and management skills, especially for clinical leaders
	Need to select "best in show" rather than "best in breed"

We now turn to findings from our interviews with leaders of civilian health care organizations and professional associations.

CHAPTER FIVE

Key Findings from Interviews with Leaders of Civilian Health Care Organizations

In this chapter, we present findings from an analysis of interviews conducted over a two-year period with 30 civilian health care executives (current and former) from 25 organizations (including nonprofit and for-profit hospitals and hospital chains, managed care organizations, and professional associations). Following the conceptual framework outlined in Chapter Two, we organize the key findings under the following broad areas: (1) context, organizational environment, and organizational leader expectations; (2) approach to leader development (i.e., how to select, how to develop, and how to incentivize); (3) the quality of the outcome, or lack thereof (i.e., the primary gaps in knowledge, skills, and abilities of medical leaders that the system needs to address); (4) challenges organizations face in identifying and developing leaders; and (5) advice or thoughts about how best to develop leaders.[1]

Note that we refer to all respondents in a gender-neutral way to ensure anonymity, but our sample included men and women.

Context, Organizational Environment, and Organizational Leader Expectations

Context and Organizational Environment

Larger organizations, such as hospital chains or integrated systems, may be more likely to have organized leadership practices.

We found that the larger systems and organizations had substantially more resources to invest in leader development and economies of scale not available to smaller systems and freestanding hospitals. In addition to having financial resources to establish internal training and education programs, larger systems also provided greater opportunities for job rotations and assignments, viewed by some executives as

---

[1] We remind the reader that we use the following terminology to characterize the number of respondents associated with a particular response: few = one or two; some = three or four; several = five to ten; many = almost all of those interviewed; and mixed = no consensus, i.e., fewer than half of those interviewed supported one view.

a valuable form of leader development.[2] Reinforcing this observation, a CEO from one of the associations stated, "Clearly, the hospitals that are in a system are typically going to have more organized leadership practices."

Many respondents in certain hospitals and systems commented on the complexity and challenges of an organizational structure in which physicians are not employed directly by the hospital or system.

Often, physicians are considered voluntary medical staff and have an elected person to represent their needs to the hospital administration. A CEO from a professional association noted that one of the things that makes health care organizations unique is that workers often have more allegiance to their profession than they do to their employing organization: "Understanding those kinds of individuals and knowing how to motivate them and [making] sure there is strategic alignment within the organization [are] important."

Similarly, a COO noted that executives have "oblique" control over physicians and that, instead of being able to "order them" to follow decisions, a leader must convince physicians based on reasoned arguments. To bridge this gap, this particular organization recently created a new collaborative council to attempt to bring senior clinical and administrative leaders together regularly to resolve issues jointly and to "incentivize" collaboration and "good behavior."

Another executive noted that this complexity pertains to all the various constituencies served by the organization. The executive explained that there were 220 categories of health care workers and 54 separate labor contracts in the organization, each with their own set of loyalties. Further, each of the various groups—whether researchers, community members, or physicians—had to feel that leaders were hearing their viewpoints. The executive believed that these demands and the different relationships of some individuals working for the organization and others operating independently created significant tension and challenges for leadership.

Respondents from health care organizations that directly employ physicians (e.g., integrated group practices) described unique structural challenges.

CEOs from several physician-led organizations noted that gaining respect and credibility among physicians is critical for leaders and that this horizontal structure required considerable courage. As one respondent explained,

> [One has] to lead an organization in which all our physicians are salaried, and the physicians follow based only and totally on the shared vision and the shared reality of what we're trying to accomplish. . . . So leaders at the very senior level have to spend a fair bit of their time doing exactly what leadership is all about, which

---

[2]   Appendix F includes examples of programs used by civilian hospitals.

is creating visions, helping to set the direction, and then sell and promote the idea and get people to really buy in.

The concept of "silos" was a prevalent theme in many interviews, and many respondents reported a need for leaders to help break down those divisions.

To illustrate, the CEO of one organization stated that "every chief has his or her own playground, and every playground has a chief administrator." The executive stated that this type of situation tends to discourage, rather than encourage, collaboration across the silos, or across the various departments and practices within the organization. In a similar vein, an association CEO discussed the notion of meta-leadership and the significance of cutting across silos. The CEO mentioned work by Harvard's Lenny Marcus in which meta-leaders achieve "connectivity," defined as a seamless web of people, organizations, resources, and information. In this context, the prefix *meta-* refers to overarching leadership that connects the purposes and the work of different organizations or organizational units (see Marcus, Dorn, and Henderson, 2005).

Two executives described intentionally structuring their organizations in ways that break down silos and make the structure more horizontal. For example, one hospital system recently reorganized from departments into cross-discipline "institutes" centered on disease and organ systems (e.g., cardiology, neurology). They had also paired clinical leaders of the institutes with administrative leaders to help with the "nuts and bolts" of the business. Centralized business capability (e.g., billing, contracting) was also said to assist leaders. These structural changes created new and different demands and expectations of leaders—most notably, interpersonal skills were at a premium. The CEO explained,

> The institute leaders have been . . . people who have interpersonal skills. Very often, you'll find . . . a department of endocrinology will be run by someone who is a great scientist. That does not make a great leader of an institute. Our Neurological Institute, for example, has 150 physicians. . . . It becomes about leadership, not about scientific acumen.

As noted earlier, the change to a horizontal structure also requires leaders to gain buy-in among physicians.

Many respondents commented on the ways in which organizational culture and environment affect leader expectations, actions, and support systems. Several interviewees identified a particular culture among physicians or physician leaders that presents challenges to leaders. One CEO commented that physicians do not like conflict and tend to think of themselves as experts and are not used to having individuals "above" them, noting that doctors have a different mindset from managers. The CEO characterized doctors as "scientific reductionists," or people who take a rigorously analytic approach to a problem and arrive at a specific solution that is "right." In the give-

and-take culture of organizations, they tend to want to prevail, and if they do not, they consider that to be "losing." Leaders, on the other hand, want to negotiate solutions that enable everyone to see him- or herself as "winning." The proclivity of doctors to see only a single solution poses challenges when they assume leadership positions. Other individuals mentioned that physician leaders tended to be "egocentric," with a lot of confidence, creating a likelihood of conflict. One executive noted an organization had to be careful about publicly identifying high-potentials for structured development efforts, because in that particular organization, all staff saw themselves as "stars."

Others commented on the ways in which the internal culture of the organization drove what they looked for and expected of leaders. For example, according to one CEO, leaders need to understand the "group thing" and how to work as a team, which was highly valued in that organization. As a result, the organization recruits people who "get this culture" and understand the dynamics of "we, not I." Similarly, another executive described an organizational culture driven by quality-improvement efforts, which emphasize that leaders do not know the answers and that everyone's goals, including those of the leaders, are to improve their work.

Finally, a few individuals commented on the external environment as a powerful influence on leader expectations in their organizations. For example, one executive noted that the organization decided it needed a different set of skills from its CEO when the health care market changed, and it recruited someone with a stronger financial background to address this new environment.

Organizational Leader Expectations

Fourteen of the 22 health care organizations had developed a specific set of leader competencies or expectations customized to their particular organizations, many of which specified expectations for executive-level leaders; others were more generic to all leaders.

In some organizations, competencies were self-developed, while others used external consultants to assist in the process. The process typically involved interviews, focus groups, and, in some cases, surveys with staff and leaders to identify either expectations for leaders or attributes of exemplary leaders. Some started with a list from an external source and modified it to fit their particular environment. Others developed the set of competencies solely from internal data.

Some of these competency models seemed to be more comprehensive in their application than others, driving multiple leader development policies and programs, such as evaluation, compensation, training, succession planning, and recruitment. Examples include the following:

- One organization's competency model involved a "success factor model" that informed training, selection, recruitment, evaluation, and compensation. These competencies were intended to establish continuity across programs and have a comprehensive influence on decisions. It consisted of four critical factors: setting direction, focusing on results, influencing others, and developing other people. As one executive noted in an article (shared with us), the competency model is invaluable in providing a framework for coming to an agreement on key behaviors for leader success and for identifying development resources and experiences for leaders at all levels.

- One of the health systems, with the assistance of an external consultant, created competency profiles for the CEO, chief financial officer (CFO), COO, and CNO, which were described in terms of business drivers. Those profiles, in turn, guided the staffing and interview process as well as development programs and would soon drive evaluations.

- Another organization had defined ten core competencies to drive evaluations, incentives, and professional development.

- Another system developed a set of "attributes and derailers" for leaders. Here, attributes included clarity of vision, communicating clearly, demonstrating a variety of leadership styles, and so on. The derailers included things like speaking negatively about members of one's department. The combination of attributes and derailers were used to drive succession planning and development activities.

- A few organizations adopted the competencies developed by the NCHL and combined them with others that were developed internally. These competencies were used to structure education and development programs, along with personnel evaluation systems.

Although some organizations referred to the HLA competencies, none adopted them outright. In fact, one of the member associations belonging to the HLA noted that these competencies were no longer relevant and that it was developing a new understanding of leadership that emphasized meta-leadership and how to lead across silos, as well as soft skills such as communication, listening, interactive approaches, and personal influence skills, which were seen to make much more of a difference than simply finance, management, and marketing.

We did not have access to all of the organizations' competencies; therefore, it is difficult to reliably summarize the content. However, some common domains included creating a vision or engaging in strategic planning, developing people, developing or managing oneself, managing resources and finance (business), promoting a culture of improvement and excellence, influencing others, and communicating or honing interpersonal skills.

The remaining eight organizations had less formal or explicit sets of expectations for leaders. Some of these organizations were in the process of developing a more formal set of competencies.

Respondents from these organizations generally gave broad answers to the question of how their organizations defined an ideal leader, such as "leaders get things done within their organizational goals," or "leaders are committed to our mission, nurturing others." Others acknowledged the value of defining competencies and explained that they were in the process of doing so.

Regardless of how formal or informal these expectations are, many organizations included both hard skills (finance, management) and soft skills (interpersonal skills, communication, building culture, inspiring others) in their conceptions of what makes a successful leader.

Several HR respondents made the distinction between skills and ability to lead on the business side (e.g., increasing operating margins, managing costs) and softer skills (e.g., building culture, inspiring and retaining staff, developing others, communicating). One CEO asserted that softer skills are most critical to achieving success and defined them as

> the ability to think about and understand where other people are coming from. It includes the ability to construct win-wins, rather than win-lose, . . . the ability to give credit and share credit, . . . the ability to effectively mentor and teach people, [and] the ability to give constructive, difficult feedback.

One HR executive noted the importance of soft skills and "influencing" skills, adding that influencing in a complex organization is tremendously important to getting things done, especially in situations in which there is little or no authority. In fact, several other executives echoed the importance of influencing skills for successful leadership. One described it as moving the organization in a desired direction through persuasion. Another described it as coaching instead of directing:

> That's a shift, because a leader doesn't know the answers. The front-line staff know the answers. You need to be able to coach and provide direction, not necessarily have the answer. . . . That's a big shift for most executive leaders as well as [those at] mid-levels.

Yet another executive called this "serving leadership" and linked it to the ability to garner support and buy-in:

> The idea . . . is that the role of the leader is to make the other people in the organization successful. . . . [It is] how you influence people to work together . . . to move the organization forward, that you really have relatively few direct control/authoritarian levers. . . . So, the ability to influence others and help others to achieve the goals through a serving mentality, without being subservient . . . becomes critical to getting people to buy in. . . . And without . . . taking time at the beginning for buy-in, it's going to be much, much more difficult to get anything done.

Stressing the importance of the soft skills, several executives asserted that these skills are not adequately taught in typical leadership programs. Others noted that interpersonal and other soft skills are difficult to teach. Conversely, several executives lamented the lack of adequate training in business skills among health care leaders. (See the section "Outcome," later in this chapter, for further discussion.)

Several executives emphasized the importance of leaders who are visionary and transformational.

"Most of all," said one former CEO, "you have to be able to formulate a strong narrative about what the future will be and be willing to face it objectively." Similarly, another explained, "When we talk to our organization about leadership, we talk about the elements of leadership. One, obviously, is having a vision about what the organization can and should be."

Yet another respondent identified the importance of transformational leadership, defined as

> identifying the new things that you want to happen, putting resources to those, and encouraging and rewarding those who do it so they become the heroes of the organization, not the people who are dragging their feet for the status quo.

Some respondents also emphasized the importance of leaders who possess strong values and moral character in addition to knowledge, skills, and abilities.

According to several CEOs, a strong values orientation is included in competency profiles for the top executives. Some examples include stewardship, integrity, and financial responsibility. One CEO noted the importance of identifying leaders with values:

> You can have the most competent person in the world, but if their values are out of sync, they will actually destroy the organization from within. So obviously, you want competency and values, but we would rather go with somebody that we could educate that has high values, rather than somebody that's really bright that has really poor values.

Similarly, another former CEO asserted that leaders need a "strong moral compass":

> The most effective health care leaders are people with very strong moral and intellectual compasses that come from deep grounding of what it is they're about and why it's important and what is moral about the way they do it. And it's from that that your wellspring of strength comes when you're trying to influence people.

A few respondents distinguished between the definition of a leader and a manager, noting that the competencies required for each are quite different.

One CEO explained that managers focus more on procedures and control, whereas leaders must be more creative:

> On the way up, you spend so much more time being a manager. You spend so much more time trying to get people to do things the right way. That's a little different than doing the right thing. . . . Managers have to be able to cope with complexity, whereas leadership has to create change, has to create the complexity. . . . Managers . . . are not the architects, but they have to build the structure. . . . Those skill sets are not the same ones you need when you're a leader. . . . And if those people can't change when they become a leader . . . you're doomed to have micromanagement; there's trouble. And micromanaging in my organization is a catastrophe.

Similarly, another CEO observed, "People mistake management and leadership." The CEO went on to eloquently describe "the art form of leadership in health care" and the importance of understanding which leadership "approach" to use for a given situation:

> It can range everywhere from . . . everybody . . . agreeing on a strategy and going from there. . . . There's . . . analytic leadership, where you're presenting as persuasive a case as you can. . . . There's what I would describe as political leadership, which is getting [influential members] engaged . . . so the organization can move forward. And then lastly, there's . . . [the] organizational terrorist. You have to be willing to . . . say, . . . "This is the way we're going," and that's very rare [but necessary] because there are times when an organization is incapable of making a decision it needs to make, just because it's too painful.

Respondents differed in their views about the importance of clinical experience and credentials for top-level executive positions.

Some respondents felt strongly that clinical experience yielded much-needed credibility. One CEO (a physician) explained that an individual gains respect in the physician community when he or she can say, "I've felt your pain." In this organization, clinical practice is expected of all leaders except the top two, and the provision of business and administrative support allows physician leaders to practice. Another CEO echoed this opinion:

> Leaders have to be concerned about what things mean to our people and our staff [and] be able to understand that. And you can't understand it if you haven't been a physician.

Others expressed more middle-ground positions. For example, one CEO (who was not a physician) believed that keeping up clinical practice was important for establishing credibility but that certain positions, such as the CEO, COO, and HR vice president, did not require a medical degree as a prerequisite. Instead, these positions require someone who gains respect from being informed:

> I think, for credibility purposes, what we have found is that those who have been most successful are those who have maintained what the body politic ultimately defines as a minimum level of competence, either clinically or academically, . . . but . . . those who have been most effective have been able to satisfy that.

Another CEO (a physician) noted that the physicians in the organization thought it was important for the CEO to be a doctor; it not only provides credibility, but it also helps doctors "deal with larger strategic moves: Somebody who was once one of them and who has felt their pain for a long time, if you will, is the one that's talking with them." However, the CEO also acknowledged that effective leaders "just won't happen by being good clinicians" and that they need more formal education and training.

Others expressed more skepticism about making the credential a prerequisite for leadership. One executive (a nonphysician) explained,

> It's a mistake to think of ultimate leadership for a clinical [individual] as necessarily being a CEO. . . . People have certain skill sets. And . . . some physicians . . . will be able to move into a CEO position. . . . It's . . . more valuable . . . to give them increasing levels of responsibility around clinical areas and [elevate] those clinical administrative responsibilities. Those are things where you want to draw on those skills, where they need that mix of clinical and managerial skills, where you can very effectively use them. . . . To have them routinely running hospitals [is not] a very good use of their skills.

Similarly, another nonphysician executive believed that "at different points in time, you need different kinds of backgrounds. . . . We're looking for talent first . . . more than background."

Approach to Leader Development

How to Select
Some respondents noted the importance of providing some common training to all executives.

One organization required all its executives to obtain 40 hours of continuing education per year. The hospital provided some opportunities to obtain this education on site, or executives could obtain it on their own outside of the organization. Another organization asked all executives to participate in its leadership program and felt that participation was important for developing a common language.

According to a hospital CEO, there are two parts to developing leaders. The first is ensuring that everyone has a common basis of understanding of the organization, decisionmaking, and accountability. The second is helping individuals grow based on their particular needs. Another executive reported that the organization developed courses for multidisciplinary groups of leaders to ensure that everyone was using a common language and also individualized opportunities for particular leaders based on interest and need.

Ten organizations had formal succession planning systems in place and deliberately sought to identify high-potentials.

These organizations generally used a similar process in which senior leaders reviewed those they supervised according to a set of criteria based on performance and potential. Many respondents referred to a "nine-box grid," used to rank individuals and identify those in the top quadrant or to assign boxes to those who demonstrated the highest performance and potential. In this process, after each senior executive rated his or her staff, the group usually came together to share and "calibrate" these ratings and discuss "top talent." Some organizations undertook this process annually; others asked senior executives to use the process to identify their own successors. In fact, one organization with rotational assignments of leaders expected each senior leader to identify three to five potential successors immediately upon accession to his or her new position.

Many organizations used this process to identify individuals who would then receive opportunities for growth and "grooming," such as mentoring or coaching, attending external programs, sitting in on board meetings, or taking on special functions or projects. At least one respondent mentioned using the process to develop low-performers, to provide these individuals with an action plan and direct them to work on areas of weakness to become at least "solid" performers or to exit the organization if they failed to improve.

According to a respondent, one organization built the process into the annual business cycle to ensure that executives saw this as part of their job and would continually think about how to identify and groom talent. This respondent also described various tools to help identify promotion, mobility, and turnover risk among these individuals.

The remaining organizations did not have formal succession planning systems in place, were in the midst of developing such a system, or had a process in place for one or two top positions. One COO voiced concerns about their organization's practice of conducting national searches for clinical leaders, calling them "academic beauty contests" that did not effectively evaluate individuals' abilities to run a business and "play nicely" with others in a collaborative way. One HR representative noted that, informally, when they found a good candidate, they tried to assign him or her projects so he or she would be less inclined to leave.

Several professional association leaders noted that succession planning was more common in larger medical centers, systems, and hospitals. They also agreed that there was growing interest in succession planning and "growing your own," which our interviews confirm.[3]

Many respondents identified hiring internal candidates as an organizational priority. According to some, internal promotion sends a message to employees that there is a future for them in the organization. Others stated a need to look externally to fill vacancies when the organization faced a crisis, such as a financial crisis or an internal conflict, in order to help "turn things around," when there is a void internally, or just to "keep it fresh."

A few executives also noted the importance of devoting attention to those who are not high-performers.

One HR representative felt that it was important to develop not only high-potentials but also "solid performers," because they are the "bread and butter" of the organization and also need opportunities for growth. Similarly, another executive noted the importance of identifying and supporting individuals who may not move into leadership positions but are critical to day-to-day operations:

> [We made] judgments about people as being high-potential, medium-potential, or well suited to their current jobs but not going anywhere above that, and we recognized that in a complex organization, you have to have a mix of the three. You can't just have high-potentials.

Available resources often drive decisions regarding whom to target for development opportunities.

An executive from a large system noted that because of that organization's size and scope, it is able to invest in future leaders, perhaps more so than smaller systems and hospitals. Two respondents noted that, given their limited budgets, the payoff was greater in providing development opportunities that apply to larger numbers of midlevel staff instead of focusing these scarce resources on a small number of top-level executives.

Several respondents considered diversity issues when deciding whom to target.

---

[3] Citing data from a report prepared for the organization, an association executive noted that, in hospitals belonging to systems—which make up 50 percent of hospitals in the country—one-quarter (26 percent) of hospital CEOs were identified in advance. This contrasted with only 15 percent of CEOs in freestanding hospitals, which make up the other 50 percent of hospitals in the country (Garman and Tyler, 2007).

One organization felt strongly that it needed to be proactive to ensure that the hospital staff reflected the community. One CEO reported that their organization had increased national and international searches for top-level positions because of the need to guarantee greater gender and ethnic diversity. One system's leadership program selected participants based, in part, on diversity of race, sex, age, and function. Similarly, another organization had implemented diversity strategies aimed to ensure that more women and minorities ended up in senior roles; in order to do so, the organization worked to develop these candidates at less senior levels to create a pipeline.

In addition to succession planning, some respondents explicitly mentioned that their organizations had an elaborate and detailed approach to the recruiting, interviewing, and hiring process for executives and considered this an important strategy for ensuring strong leaders.

Several executives reported using behavioral interview questions to identify individuals who possessed the competencies and behaviors they sought in their leaders, while others mentioned specific screening techniques to assess individuals' values. One such hospital had 150 behavioral interview questions available to adapt when hiring for specific positions. One CEO believed that behavioral interviewing ensured strong leadership because it is better to find someone "built of the right stuff" and teach him or her how to do the job. In their book, Leonard Berry and Kent Seltman describe management practices at the Mayo Clinic, explaining that one of that organization's characteristics—and among characteristics of high-performing organizations in general—is deliberative hiring, involving screening and behavioral interviews by panels of staff. The authors explain,

> The essential element . . . is the value set from which the spontaneous service flows; kindness and humanely sensitive acts come more reliably from underlying values than from training sessions. . . . Mayo Clinic, like other high-performing service organizations, takes particular care in identifying people's values before they are hired. (Berry and Seltman, 2008, p. 154)

Others mentioned recruitment strategies intended to attract individuals who would be effective in their organizations. For example, one former CEO noted the importance of hiring some individuals from outside of the organization because these "outsiders" could be innovative and bring in ideas about "what the organization can be." Another organization routinely recruited doctors immediately out of clinical training programs to ensure a willingness to participate as members of a team and group practice and felt that individuals who had been out of their training for more than five years no longer "get the group thing." This same organization also allowed for part-time employment as a means to attract "wonderful physicians" who would not otherwise practice if they had to work full time (e.g., women with young children). This organization found that as these physicians matured, these part-time employees generally increased their hours and their hours devoted to leadership, thereby allowing the organization to adapt to individual needs while also investing in future leaders.

How to Develop

Not all activities described in this section are discrete—that is, some integrate coaching or mentoring with formal education and with on-the-job assignments. A good example of this is a large system's COO development program (which primarily falls under training and education but includes elements of other types of activities).

Overall Approach. Respondents noted varied approaches to leader development across their organizations, including team leader development and individualized activities. Some also noted that the industry is not doing a good job in developing leaders.

Some organizations described the need for cross-functional and customized approaches to professional development, including team leader development.

According to one executive, providing cross-functional or interdisciplinary opportunities helps to cut across silos within organizations. For clinical leaders, this would entail identifying what roles outside of one's clinical discipline he or she needs to take on and is suited for, and then finding ways to develop the skills and knowledge needed to take on these roles. Two other organizations emphasized cross-functional participation in *team* leader development activities. For example, two organizations participated in the Leadership Excellence Networks (LENS) sponsored by the NCHL,[4] which explicitly requires participating teams to include individuals from different areas of the organization. One participating executive explained,

> We also try to make sure that we mix different . . . kinds of people with different perspectives on these [LENS] teams so that they get an opportunity to . . . walk in somebody else's shoes. . . . You might take . . . a person from the health plan who's been frustrated [and] give that person an opportunity to work on the other side in the delivery system. . . . And you take somebody in the delivery system who never has trusted the health plan and you give them a chance to work in the health plan and understand what their challenges are. . . . Everybody . . . comes back, if nothing else, a lot more cooperative than they ever were before.

---

[4]   According to the NCHL, LENS

joins organizations together that are committed to developing, adopting, and sharing leading practices and new knowledge. Through collaboration and leveraging our cutting-edge research and tools, organizations can strengthen their leadership capabilities, driving systematic and sustainable changes. (NCHL, undated)

LENS includes so-called "C-suite" leaders—e.g., CEOs, COOs, CFOs, CNOs—and provides opportunities for these leaders to share best practices in leadership development and related initiatives.

Some respondents also highlighted the importance of customizing development opportunities based on where individuals are in terms of their development. One organization, for example, provided staff with a "stair-step" series of development opportunities based on their experience and developmental level.

According to one HR representative,

> When developing leaders, organizations should consider team development and how people work together. This organization is interviewing the executive team to identify what they want to work on and assess how effective they are at communicating with each other, etc.—then bringing in consultants.

Another CEO described focusing on team development and meeting with the management team regularly to challenge its members to "problem-solve as a group and learn a collaborative dynamic instead of an individual dynamic."

Other organizations created specific team-based development programs for top-level leaders. For example, one organization nominated administrator and physician pairs to attend its parent-company leader development program, because it was viewed as a best practice among high-performing organizations. Others invited larger groups of executives to participate in professional development. One former executive described a past team-focused leadership program (since discontinued) that was perceived to be effective in developing softer leadership skills and exposing individuals to diverse perspectives. "This approach to bringing various disciplines together," the executive said, "begin[s] to [give] an appreciation for what each other brought to the table. So the finance people or the organizational people had administrative skills that the physicians needed to get what they wanted [out of the program]." The teams' focus on real projects was also believed to enhance the effects of these development opportunities:

> It's also an opportunity to educate people and bring them along to a place they may not have thought they would ever get before because of the power of the group, and of the discussion, and of the information.

Some respondents believed that it was important to provide a blend of common and individualized development activities, which may include internal and external opportunities.

In addition to "common development activities," which help provide a common language and promote collaboration across disciplines, some organizations also offered individualized activities to ensure alignment with particular needs and interests. In fact, many executives seemed to agree that, for top talent at the most senior levels, individualized support was needed most. For example, one organization created personal development plans for leaders and high-potentials based on formal and 360-degree evaluations to identify specific needs and customized development opportunities. "It all depends on what the deficit is," this organization's executive explained.

Sometimes we can solve that from inside; sometimes we can solve that with a different assignment inside. And sometimes we have to send somebody to a specific course that seems to do a good job of dealing with that particular problem or issue or deficiency.

As noted earlier, another organization developed courses for multidisciplinary groups of leaders to ensure that everyone was using a common language. It also provided individualized opportunities for particular leaders based on interest and need. One professional association executive described an ideal mix of providing leaders with internal development opportunities to focus on broad leadership issues—and their application to the specific organization—and external opportunities to provide interaction with individuals from other settings. Other executives identified the value of providing leaders with opportunities not only to exchange ideas with individuals from other organizations with different perspectives on how to address problems but also to learn from fields outside of health care.

In fact, LENS, to which Henry Ford and Trinity belong, explicitly fosters information exchange across organizations in its leader development programs. One Henry Ford executive (not interviewed but cited in documents collected for this study) noted,

> One of the important values of LENS is the ability to share learnings with other organizations in a safe environment. . . . Understanding what has worked elsewhere and creating pilots around those successes has important value to us because [of the] cost savings and the efficiencies that it creates. (NCHL, 2006, p. 3)

Similarly, an executive from Trinity (also not interviewed) noted,

> LENS provides a unique opportunity for healthcare organizations to benchmark themselves using NCHL's research and outcomes. LENS senior executives have the opportunity to share ideas in a peer-to-peer setting, to reflect on them, and then share their experiences and outcomes from implementation in their organizations. . . . LENS provides a platform for organizations that are looking for companionship in leadership formation. (NCHL, 2008, p. 2)

As an overall assessment of development activities, a few executives noted that the industry is either doing a terrible job or simply waits too long in the leader's career to provide support.

One individual believed that many organizations tend to offer newly selected executives a "survival skills" course that often occurs too late in their careers. An HR representative agreed with this assessment and believed that her organization had not been purposeful in how it approached professional development. This executive noted that her organization often sent executives to a course without asking why or what the individual or organization would get out of it in return and did not connect the development activity to the organization's strategic priorities. Similarly, others observed that executives in health care organizations often avoided conflict and did not take early steps to identify individuals' needs and problems and to develop their skills.

We now discuss respondents' views on the specific leader development strategies outlined in the conceptual framework in Chapter Two.

Job Assignments and Experiences. Like the military respondents, civilian health care executives emphasized the value of on-the-job experience. Civilian organizations took a variety of approaches to providing these opportunities to potential leaders.

Several respondents emphasized the need for experiential and applied learning opportunities.

Citing anecdotal evidence, one HR executive stated that 70 percent of managers' growth comes from hands-on experience, 20 percent from coaching, and 10 percent from in-class learning. Reinforcing this, another HR representative stated that learning at the executive level comes less from formal training and more from developmental assignments and on-the-job training. Another executive ascribed to the notion of "time, space, learning," in which individuals experiment with what they learn from training or educational opportunities, have the space to apply what they learn in their jobs, and then come back to discuss it. Similarly, an executive from another organization identified applied projects as the most powerful form of development:

> If you're giving someone a stretch assignment, for example, then you would work with them closely on it and help them, be an adviser behind the scenes, helping them work through it. . . . If not by volume, in terms of meaningfulness, our most powerful development is in that kind of applied way.

An association executive believed that emerging leaders needed incremental opportunities to apply what they learned, as opposed to a single training experience, which may or may not be reinforced.

Job rotations occurred in five organizations.

Although one association leader noted that formal job rotations are rare in health care organizations, five organizations in our sample employed some form of this practice. Well known for institutionalizing this practice, the Mayo Clinic keeps most leaders in their positions from five to ten years before rotating them to other positions in which they keep whatever salary adjustment they had earned. The executive explained that the rotation of leadership helps foster teamwork, eliminates any power bases that might develop when one individual stays in a leadership position indefinitely, and creates incentives for positive leadership behavior because those in current leadership positions realize that, in the future, they will be led by the individuals they are now leading. Rotation on and off of various committees for two- to three-year periods was also viewed as a means of developing a pipeline for future leaders, providing individuals with exposure to a broad base of knowledge about the dynamics of the organization.

At Virginia Mason, high-level executives who are being developed as leaders are assigned to two-year positions in what that organization calls the Kaizen Promotion Office to "learn deeply" the methodology of improvement promoted by the Toyota Production System and to gain exposure to other parts of the organization. These individuals are expected to work with executives to improve the performance of "flow and value streams," to lead workshops and other activities, and to "manage changes" to ensure that they are implemented.

According to our respondents, a few other large systems also intentionally "move people around" to give them a variety of organizational experiences and perspectives.

Thirteen of the 22 organizations assigned short-term projects as a means of exposing leaders and potential leaders to multiple facets of the organization and providing them with opportunities to try out new skills and apply new knowledge.

Many organizations believed that projects and committee assignments were important, especially for cutting across potential "silos" that may exist in the organization. For example, as part of its talent-review process, one organization identified short-term project assignments for individuals needing development in a particular area. Examples cited included leading a project on consolidation or standardizing clinical education practice, participating as a group member in purchasing a new piece of software, or participating in a project aimed at opening a new freestanding ambulatory clinic. Another organization had a "top ten project list" based on the strategic priorities that it assigned to top performers and directors or managers whom it did not want to lose. Similarly, another organization's physician leadership program included projects that involved participants in areas outside of their own expertise. An executive from another organization described giving high-potentials stretch assignments to help develop their skills. As noted earlier, many executives felt that these hands-on projects were extremely powerful development opportunities.

Respondents from several organizations also mentioned the assignment of individuals to various committees as yet another means of allowing them to learn about the organization more broadly than would be the case from working in their one department or area.

One organization expressed an interest in job assignments ("developmental assignments") as part of its new development system for high-performers. Interestingly, one organization was working with external consultants and a business unit in the system to create a program that allowed one person the opportunity to try out a position for a few months and then return to his or her original position. One HR executive asserted that it is important to give potential leaders experiential knowledge and the opportunity to experience the incumbent's job.

A few organizations paired physician leaders with administrative managers to facilitate team leadership.

For example, at the Mayo Clinic, administrative leaders are assigned to work as partners with physician leaders (e.g., an operations administrator paired with the chair of cardiology) to enhance leadership of the hospital. The chief administrative officer of its Arizona facility is quoted in a book about the clinic, stating that "high-quality management decisions emerge from the healthy tension between the patient-first advocacy of the physician leader and advocacy for fiscal responsibility from the administrator" (Berry and Seltman, 2008, p. 103). The executive goes on to say,

> Physicians are educated to act creatively and independently with a focus on best serving the individual patient. The administrators are trained to apply concepts of managerial and organization theory, to foster group performance, and to provide systems and procedures that enable patient satisfaction, quality, and financial success. Effective administration will aggregate information and will help doctors look at the bigger picture—groups of patients or department operational statistics rather than lab values for the individual patient. (p. 104)

Leaders at Mayo acknowledge, however, that the success of this approach depends in large part on the "art" of making a good match between these two individuals.

Education and Training. Almost all organizations offered some kind of education or training to staff, either internally or externally.

Many organizations sponsored internal courses and educational opportunities for staff.

Some health care systems have their own "university" or "academy" where they offer courses on a range of leadership and management topics to all staff. Some organizations develop courses and opportunities on their own, while others work with consultants or purchase programs from vendors, such as the Advisory Board Company, or through professional associations.

Some organizations have designed leader development programs specifically for middle managers. For example, Beth Israel has a program that generally runs four hours a week for 18 months and is designed for middle managers viewed as having the potential to rise to senior leadership positions. The program, which is said to be "transformational," pairs all participants with a senior-level mentor; provides training in presentation skills, how to lead meetings, and other topics; and involves participants in project-based assignments. As a different approach, Vanderbilt's Leadership Development Institute is a full-day session held quarterly for all managers.

In addition to the types of programs noted here, some are focused exclusively on executives or clinical leaders. Specific examples are provided in Appendix F. These range from a three- to four-day advanced leadership program to a three- to five-year experience involving a cohort of around 45 individuals. Most of these programs involve projects, structured learning, and, sometimes, an internship. Often, there is a self-assessment and coaching component. In addition, several organizations sponsor retreats for top leaders, which serve as both a strategic planning activity for the organization and a development opportunity for individuals. The specific development opportunities aimed at clinical leaders often involve case studies and experiential learning targeted at improving business and management skills.

Almost all of the organizations sponsored external professional development and educational opportunities for leaders.

An executive from a professional association stated that in freestanding hospitals and smaller systems, it is more typical to send people outside of the organization for professional development activities. Most commonly, organizations sponsored individuals with high potential to attend external training and or educational sessions. Because these programs tend to be expensive, some organizations maximized the return on their investments by asking participants to conduct projects for the organization after completing the program or course. One respondent said that this was a good way to sustain the learning for participants and add value for the organization. Many organizations pay the tuition for individuals to obtain advanced degrees. Some examples are provided in Appendix F.

A few executives, however, questioned the value of some of these external leader development programs. One individual noted that some of these courses often do not "add up to a course of study." Another cautioned, "We don't believe in any of these 14-day-wonder kind of programs, where we send you to Harvard for two weeks and you're going to be a star. We don't believe in that."

Mentoring and Coaching. As in the military, informal mentoring or coaching was very common in civilian health care organizations. Unlike the military, many organizations employed coaches to facilitate leader development.

Executive coaching (externally provided) was more widespread than formal mentoring.

An association CEO stated that formal mentoring was not common in hospitals and health care systems because it is often difficult for people to stay together for a long time. Other respondents noted that coaching from an external source was often needed for top-level executives who, given their level of responsibility and privileged knowledge, could not turn to internal mentors for assistance and needed a more confidential, third-party mentor.

One large system's leader development program paired each participant with a CEO mentor. Although this organization planned to add more structure to the process, the current mentor-mentee relationship involved each party signing a member agreement to meet regularly. One noted challenge with this arrangement was that the CEO was both mentor and manager.

One hospital, which had one of the few formal mentoring programs geared toward nonclinical managers (such as business-unit managers), provided some training to mentors and those being mentored. In this arrangement, the mentored were paired with someone outside of their department to demonstrate how different areas of the system worked together (not in "silos"). There were mixed views regarding its effectiveness.

Many respondents mentioned the existence of informal mentoring that occurs naturally within the organization.

A leader of an association felt strongly that one cannot "assign mentorship" but instead could assign people to assist. This executive noted that individuals seek out their mentors and that organizations could not formally institute these relationships. Other executives explained that mentoring is expected of all leaders. Some, however, acknowledged that these responsibilities are often cast aside when more urgent demands arise. One leader described mentoring as a "coming-and-going phenomenon":

> So you have this constant battle between your mentoring and developmental responsibilities as a leader and just the demands of day-in, day-out, getting things done or the crises that you face. Health care is nothing if not a crisis-oriented kind of environment. . . . So, when things are calm, you'll see people spending a lot of time mentoring and . . . [focusing] on development plans.

Many organizations employed coaches—primarily external consultants—to assist executives with development.

At one organization, coaches were available on a voluntary basis to individuals who are having trouble with a particular issue or who are high-performers seeking to move up in the organization. Another hospital employed coaches to help executives with particular issues or problems. Here, the HR representative reported that there were two "executive consultants" for senior vice presidents and above, describing them as "partly remedial," used to help "straighten executives out" or keep them out of trouble.

While some organizations used coaches to help leaders who were having trouble, others employed them more proactively to develop leader skills. In one large system, coaching was used mostly as a form of development, and those who had used the coaches often described this as the most valuable development opportunity they encountered. The system's HR leaders were trying to identify best vendors and best practices to help facilitate this process.

Follow-up coaching was embedded in one organization's leader development programs to ensure the application and transfer of knowledge. That organization used external coaches and was trying to build internal capacity but found it difficult, in particular, to gain access to the "real vulnerabilities" of leaders.

Some organizations had a range of coaches available to leaders. For example, at one hospital, "lean" coaches and quality coaches acted as internal resources for middle managers to help out with a specific issue for six-week periods, whereas external coaches were available to executives only and were intended to help them prepare for a promotion or large project.

One respondent noted that the confidentiality offered by an external coach was extremely important for executives who often could not turn to internal sources. At another organization, coaches were used to assist with follow-up steps after the 360-degree evaluation process, helping individuals develop growth plans and find resources to implement them.

Career Counseling and Feedback. Although we did not obtain much information on this topic, the one activity that was mentioned repeatedly was the use of voluntary evaluations and feedback on performance.

Many organizations were using 360-degree evaluations and personal development plans to facilitate development opportunities, although how these were used appeared to vary based on who was being targeted.

For example, at one hospital, all executives, directors, and managers were doing 360-degree evaluations for development purposes, allowing them to see how peers and supervisors perceive them. The report goes only to the employee being reviewed, and he or she then has the option of bringing in coaches to help with development. This organization was adamant about not making the report part of the formal evaluation, instead encouraging individuals to develop growth plans that could be shared with a supervisor. The leader explained,

> We want employees to feel very comfortable recognizing that this is a [professional development] process, [that] they are not being evaluated on it and nothing negative will come of it, but, rather, we want them to continue to grow and develop.

Other organizations similarly involved leaders in creating personal development, growth, or learning plans to address the various needs identified by these assessments. One executive was adamant that the process of developing a learning plan based on 360-degree feedback was intended to spur real growth and development: "It wasn't about taking another course. It was about action."

Self-Development. Self-development was less common among civilian organizations than in the military.

The majority of organizations did not cite self-development as an important component of their leader development approach.

As noted earlier, the respondents we interviewed reported that their organizations sponsored other types of activities and did not simply leave it up to individual executives to seek out support. Nevertheless, several respondents noted that executives often already had strong technical skills and frequently participated in and were encouraged to participate in external conferences and association-related development opportunities to add to their knowledge and skills in areas of particular interest.

How to Incentivize

Every organization involved top executives in some form of annual performance-based evaluation. These processes tended to emphasize evaluation based on measurable metrics that were tied to broader organizational goals as well as to individual goals, and they were generally linked to incentive or compensation plans based on weighted formulas.

According to the leader of one association, most executives were on contracts, and they were most likely evaluated on organizational performance (e.g., finance, employee measures), followed by quality and then professional responsibility.

Some organizations seemed to focus exclusively on outcomes and measurable objectives (e.g., relative value units, which measure, on a common scale, the resources needed to provide specific services and ensure patient satisfaction, safety, and quality, for example). While most evaluation systems evaluate what leaders accomplish over the year, some also assess how they have accomplished their goals. The "how" tends to be guided by leadership competencies, described by some as the "nonmeasurables," such as how an individual develops others or handles HR issues. For example, in one organization that emphasized the "what" and "how," the annual performance evaluation equally weighed measures of what (50 percent) and how (50 percent).

In many organizations, somewhat separate goals were assessed on an individual's annual evaluation, and then a subset of those goals was factored into the incentive or compensation plan. A few respondents noted that evaluations in their organizations were based in part on self-assessments, along with input from peers and supervisors.

A handful of respondents noted the importance of rewards and recognition for leaders and emerging leaders—rewards that were not necessarily financial.

One executive emphasized the importance of rewards and recognition, whether it be a supervisor sending a letter to someone he or she sees as having done a good job or standing out as a leader, or providing those with demonstrated talent or accomplishments a special title and project to take on. For example, this organization named "physician champions" in various areas of interest. The executive explained,

I'll call them and say, "What excites you to come to work—other than clinical practice? . . . You're now physician champion of whatever excites you, and here's a little bit of time to do it, here's a couple extra dollars if you succeed." . . . Rewards and recognition at every level are just so important. I think the military has it down. . . . They have . . . institutionalized ways of recognizing and moving people on. [Interviewer: But you might get the title of physician champion?] Yes, physician champion, assistant chief of —, director, physician director of — . . . is an implicit reward, and then at some point, somebody genuinely recognizes you financially. . . . But the power of a letter from the person above you, or the power of a letter to your boss [is great], and that costs nothing. I've got people framing these letters and putting them on their mantelpieces.

One HR representative described the organization's "leadership week," which included not only speakers and activities for development, but also recognition of accomplishments (although this seemed to target lower-level leaders).

Some respondents noted that inviting individuals to participate in selected professional development programs is a form of recognition in and of itself, signaling that the organization sees their potential and wants to invest in their future. As one executive said, "We showcased this leadership training as a real investment in people and something that people would be very proud of having been selected for."

A few organizations seemed to be using evaluation systems to build a "culture of professional development expectation."

Some organizations created an expectation that individuals participate in ongoing education and training. One organization's new evaluation system required all executives to acquire 40 hours of continuing education each year to become eligible for pay increases. Similarly, an executive at another organization that also required at least 40 hours of education per year stated, "I think it helps when you say, 'This is what we expect.'" We heard of only one organization that provided bonuses to executives who became ACHE fellows (which requires passing an exam to become board-certified).

Outcome

Respondents in almost every organization commented on potential weaknesses in the knowledge, skills, and experience of current clinical leaders.

Sometimes, the topic simply came up unsolicited; at other times, we asked a direct question about executives in general and whether there were certain areas in which executives were weak or needed more support. Notably, most respondents tended to focus on clinical leaders. Many stated that these leaders were often promoted because they were excellent clinicians, which did not necessarily transfer into good leadership skills. One association CEO stated that organizations cannot assume that expert clinicians will "blossom into having leadership skills with no work." The perceived weaknesses or areas of need generally fit into two broad categories: interpersonal and financial and business management.

Interpersonal. One CEO stated that clinicians often have weaknesses in personnel management, understanding organizational and group dynamics in complex organizations, and using people effectively. Further, this executive believed that physicians are often good in small groups but that talent does not always "scale up."

Another CEO asserted that clinicians need better supervisory and people skills, especially in terms of how to deal with the emotional issues that employees bring to a manager, how not to condescend, and how to balance being in charge with not "bossing people." A COO felt that cultural competence was a major shortcoming of clinical leaders: understanding interpersonal nuances, managing in a diverse environment, and being able to lead with professionalism and use empathy to empower people who may be of different backgrounds. An HR executive noted that clinical leaders are weaker on the softer skills—building high-performing teams, culture, and vision; empowering people; and exercising emotional intelligence—which are more difficult to teach than the business side of leadership.

As noted earlier, another CEO described how physicians tend to have uncompromising and absolute views, and cannot negotiate win-win situations but instead seek win-lose situations. This executive also commented that clinicians do not like conflict, tend to think of themselves as experts, and are not used to having individuals above them. Several other executives similarly observed that health care leaders tend to be "conflict avoiders" who often do not know how to coach a person toward improvement or move people out of positions when they are simply not fit for the job. An association CEO noted that clinicians need help with the relationship side of leadership—getting people to work together and breaking down silos—which tends to be harder to teach than the business side. Another association CEO stated that most clinical leaders grow disengaged because of shortcomings in interpersonal skills: "Success in the field depends 90 percent on interpersonal skills and 10 percent [on] technical skills."

Financial and Business Management. In addition to the softer skills, which seemed to be much more critical to the leaders we interviewed, many executives also stated that clinical leaders tend to lack necessary abilities in finance, decision science, managing large and complex systems, supply chain management, and IT familiarity. One executive noted that training programs do not adequately equip health care leaders with project management, quality improvement, and process mapping skills.

Other Comments on Improving Leader Development

Respondents from many organizations commented on the importance of supporting leader development at the highest level.

One executive stated that board buy-in is critical to the talent management and development process, and the organization should "not just give it lip service." This includes investing in infrastructure resources and making a commitment to managing the process of identifying potential leaders. Another executive believed that the organization needs to decide that "leadership is as important as anything they can do."

Some respondents noted the importance of having a solid competency model as the basis for leader development.

An executive of a large system stated that an organization must have a solid competency model that people buy into, have agreement that executives will then hire and place graduates of internal programs intended to groom individuals, ensure executive sponsorship of programs, and ensure transparency of programs or otherwise risk engendering mistrust.

Many respondents commented on the need for effective hiring processes and the need to be purposeful when interviewing for executive positions.

For example, one organization used a behavioral-based approach and looked at past performance to determine whether there was a good fit. One executive raised the idea of requiring leaders to develop a portfolio demonstrating how they have improved their skills each year and using it as the basis for promotions. Instead of promoting individuals because "they are in the right place at the right time," this leader suggested asking individuals to demonstrate the experiences they have had, the types of problems they have solved, and the challenges they have faced.

Several respondents identified the importance of mentoring and coaching.

One stated that executive coaching should be used not just when someone has a problem but also to help prepare someone for a promotion or a large project. Another executive believed that coaches were critical for top-level leader development tailored to individual needs:

> At the most executive level, individual coaches would be critical. And to really target the learning around specific issues that they're struggling with. And they don't want to struggle in public. . . . If I went to an individual group, I would say everyone should be required to have a coach. Everyone needs to learn. But what they need to learn is very different.

As discussed earlier, experiential and individualized activities were frequently mentioned as key leader development activities.

Several respondents emphasized that "we learn by doing." One explained, "I do believe it's 30 percent learning and 70 percent applying, and that the process allows for integration of what I'm learning into practice in a safe environment."

Development activities should expose leaders or potential leaders to different viewpoints and perspectives. For example, one executive advised that leaders in one type of organization could learn from the activities and practices of other types of organizations:

> [I advise] exposing people as much as possible to different organizations and different ways of looking at things, or different ways of doing things, because it helps to understand a broad range of possibilities. . . . We can do that because we're big enough and complex enough. We can move people from area to area, and they can get very different viewpoints.

Finally, a few executives advocated for leader development in health care to focus more on process control and improvement, such as the concepts from Toyota manufacturing.

One CEO attested to the value gained personally from studying these ideas and strategies, which helped the CEO "think beyond my confines as a general surgeon."

Summary of Findings from Interviews

Table 5.1 summarizes the views of civilian leaders with respect to the main categories of leader development.

Table 5.1
Overview of Themes Identified in Interviews with Civilian Leaders

Area	Findings
Context and organizational environment	Organized approach to leader development more likely at larger organizations
	Gaining credibility with and cooperation of physicians (especially those not directly employed by the hospital) seen as challenging
	Need to break down "silos" stressed by many
Organizational leader expectations	Specific sets of leader competencies or expectations developed by many organizations, although some adopted less formal approaches
	Both "hard" and "soft" skills recognized as necessary for leaders
	Being visionary and transformational mentioned as important by several
	Values and character seen by some as important
	Distinction between a leader and a manager emphasized by some
	Mixed views on need for leaders to possess and maintain clinical skills

Table 5.1—Continued

Area	Findings
Approach to leader development	Strategic, purposeful approach to selection and development adopted by some (see "How to select" and "How to develop")
How to select:	Need for common training for all executives stressed by some
Succession planning	Formal succession plans that seek to identify employees with high potential adopted by some
Formal strategies, including screening, behavioral interviews, and targeted recruiting	Need to attend to those who are the "bread and butter" of the organization (in addition to the high-performers) mentioned by some
	Development opportunities sometimes limited by availability of resources
	Attention to diversity when deciding whom to target mentioned as an important criterion by several
	Detailed and structured approach to recruiting personnel mentioned by some, including screening and behavioral interviews by panels of staff and recruiting targeted at individuals who might "fit" with the organization

How to develop: Job assignments Other development opportunities Education and training Mentoring and coaching Career counseling and feedback	Purposeful development strategies adopted by some, including
	    Cross-functional development (seen as important to break down silos)
	    Individualized development opportunities based on personal development plans and/or 360-degree evaluations
	    Common training for multidisciplinary groups of leaders to ensure common language
	    Providing leader development for teams

	Some concerns mentioned by a few (slowness in providing career development support or lack of connection between development courses and organization's strategic priorities)
	Consensus regarding the importance of job assignments and the need for experiential and applied learning opportunities (for example, job rotations, short-term projects, teaming physicians and administrators)
	Internal educational opportunities offered by many; external development opportunities supported by almost all

	External coaching more widespread than formal mentoring
	    Widely used for high-level executive development
	    Informal mentoring widespread

	Use of voluntary 360-degree evaluations, feedback, and personal development plans mentioned by several
	Self-development not seen as an important development component
How to incentivize: Performance-based evaluations Monetary and nonmonetary rewards and recognition	Annual performance evaluation with emphasis on measurable metrics tied to broader organizational goals Incentive plans linked to organizational goals
	Nonmonetary rewards and recognition seen as important
	Ongoing participation in education and training required by some for pay increases
Outcome	Critical of leadership, business, and management skills of clinical leaders (including interpersonal skills)

This chapter examined how civilian health care organizations identify, develop, and evaluate leaders for executive positions. We now turn our attention to the government sector and examine how the VHA approaches leader development.

CHAPTER SIX

Case Study: The Veterans Health Administration's Approach to Leader Development

Over the past several years, the Veterans Health Administration (VHA) has spent considerable time and effort in developing and implementing a leader development program, including a workforce-development and succession plan that has been recognized by the Office of Personnel Management as a federal best practice (VA, 2009a). Since the VHA is both a high-performing medical health system and a government agency, we hypothesized that a more extensive analysis would give us deeper insight into what made it such a successful operation only about a decade after it was widely criticized for poor management. As was the case with the military and civilian groups, we interviewed senior managers. We conducted 16 interviews with senior leaders at the VHA, five of whom were network and facility directors; the remainder were central office (VHACO) leaders involved in leader development programs, evaluation, and organizational learning. However, we broadened our inquiry at the VHA to include a more extensive contextual analysis and documentary reviews of its policies for selecting, developing, and promoting members of the staff, including competencies developed.

We should note that the information presented here was current as of spring 2009. A senior leader in the VHA noted recently that the organization is undergoing significant transformation under the new VA and VHA leadership, including the launching of a comprehensive human capital initiative to make the VA a "veteran- and people-centric, results-oriented, and forward-looking organization."[1] As part of this effort, the VHA is evaluating its current leader development programs to ensure that they meet and further the goals of the organization's new leadership. As a result, the competency model that underpins the leadership programs described herein may be changing.

Note that we refer to all interview respondents in a gender-neutral way to ensure anonymity, but our sample included men and women.

The U.S. Department of Veterans Affairs (VA) was established as an independent agency in 1930 under President Herbert Hoover by Executive Order 5398 and elevated to Cabinet level in 1989 by Public Law 100-527. The VA has three major line organiza-

---

[1] Personal communication, April 4, 2010.

tions: the VHA, Veterans Benefits Administration, and National Cemetery Administration. Each of these agencies reports to the Secretary of Veterans Affairs through the Deputy Secretary. Each administration has a Washington, D.C.–based central office that directs the administration's operations and gives centralized program direction to the field facilities that provide program services to veterans and their families.

With more than 235,000 employees, the VHA is the third-largest civilian employer in the federal government and one of the largest providers of health care in the world. It is the nation's largest integrated health care delivery system and provides care through 21 Veterans Integrated Service Networks (VISNs) distributed throughout the United States.

The next several sections discuss (1) the context and organizational environment of the VHA, (2) leader expectations as embodied in the VHA's High Performance Development Model (HPDM), and (3) the organization's approach to leader development—including selection and development strategies as evidenced by selected leader development programs and feedback to individuals through the evaluation process. Because evaluation of programs is strongly emphasized by the VHA, we discuss this topic in a separate section. A final section summarizes advice or comments from interviewees about specific leader development issues.

Context, Organizational Environment, and Organizational Leader Expectations

Context and Organizational Environment

Transformation of the VHA. The VA—and the VHA in particular—has undergone a remarkable transformation. As Perlin, Kolodner, and Roswell (2004, p. 829) note,

> In the late 1980s and early 1990s, the VA was beset by increasing public anxiety about the quality of care. A 1992 movie titled *Article 99*, made in Hollywood by Orion Pictures, parodied the VA as a hapless and dangerous bureaucracy, and the challenging US economy at the close of the 1980s and opening of the next decade raised concern about the economic viability of the system. . . . [A] tension emerged between the desire to maintain a system dedicated to veterans' health needs and vouchering out (contracting for) care for presumably greater quality and efficiency. It was increasingly apparent that if the VA were to survive, it would need to prove its value to Congress and its quality to veterans themselves.

Then–Under Secretary for Health Kenneth Kizer described the challenges facing the VA in two landmark documents, *Vision for Change* and *Prescription for Change* (Kizer, 1995, 1996), which served as the basis for the structural and organizational reinvention of VHA.

This reinvention mandated structural and organizational changes, rationalization of resource allocation, measurement and active management of quality and value (and clear accountability for quality and value), and an information infrastructure that would increasingly support the needs of patients, clinicians, and administrators. . . .

The structural changes were predicated on the assumption that providing the most effective, efficient care required coordination among facilities and synergy of resources, including that care be provided in the most appropriate environments. (Perlin, Kolodner, and Roswell, 2004, pp. 828–829)

The restructuring led to the creation of 22 (now 21) geographically determined VISNs, which were given control over the medical centers, community-based outpatient clinics, long-term care facilities, and other programs in each region. Resources were reallocated to each network and depend on the number and complexity of unique cases served at each facility. Each VISN is led by a network director who operates under a performance contract with the VHA Under Secretary for Health. This contract, in turn, cascades down to clinicians and managers throughout the system. This subject is discussed in more detail later in this chapter. Results of the performance contract are reviewed quarterly and are widely available. The VA describes this process as a bold move to decentralize the VHA's bureaucracy, eliminate layers of administration, bring staff closer to patient care, and ensure accountability.

Fundamentally, VHA transformed itself from a collection of "safety net" hospitals to a health system focused on health promotion and disease prevention. . . .

Restructuring our organization was just the beginning. We needed a way to hold ourselves accountable for making quality and safety non-negotiable standards for Veterans' care. So we began to quantify care delivery with an aggressive use of performance measurements for field and headquarters managers. These measurements have led to a consistent application of evidence-based guidelines that systemize the best practices in government and private-sector care. (U.S. Department of Veterans Affairs, 2009b, p. 8)

The hard work, time, and effort devoted to transformation seem to have paid off. A 2003 study, the results of which were published in the *New England Journal of Medicine*, found that the VHA performed "significantly better" on 11 quality measures than fee-for-service Medicare providers (Jha et al., 2003). A RAND study showed that the VA outperformed U.S. health care organizations in other sectors on a comprehensive list of quality indicators (Asch et al., 2004). Patients receiving care from the VA have reported higher levels of satisfaction than patients receiving care in the private sector (Ibrahim, 2007). According to surveys by the National Quality Research Center at the University of Michigan, for more than six years, the VA has received the highest consumer satisfaction ratings of any public- or private-sector health care system. The success it has achieved over the past decade has been attributed to several factors: strong leadership development, transition from a hospital-based system to an integrated health care system, creation of regionally financed health care through VISNs, introduction of performance-based incentives for competition, and the development of the electronic health record (Oliver, 2008). Others highlight the systematic use of data-driven measures to monitor performance across several domains, including technical quality of care, access, functional status, and patient satisfaction (Kerr and Fleming, 2007).

A significant part of the transformation of the VHA has been the attention paid to leader and workforce development throughout the organization.

We discuss this topic in the next several sections. The next section briefly describes the organizational structure that was set up to ensure collaboration across the various offices of the VHA and, most particularly, input from the field with respect to leader development and organizational improvement.

VHA Organizational Structure. The VHA's overall governance body is the National Leadership Board (NLB), chaired by the Under Secretary for Health.[2] Its members include all top-level senior executives in the VHA, including the 21 VISN directors and the heads of all major health care program offices at VHA headquarters. A smaller executive committee consisting of ten members of the NLB is largely responsible for day-to-day decisionmaking. Several committees oversee the major health care and business areas of the organization, as shown in Figure 6.1. The Succession and Workforce Development Management Subcommittee is a standing subcommittee of the HR Committee of the NLB, as is the Organizational Assessment Subcommittee. These two subcommittees work closely on workforce development and succession programs, "with an expertise and emphasis on workplace improvement, employee satisfaction, and organizational development research." As the plan further notes,

> Having a permanent, accountable organization linked directly to the top VHA leadership structure, to oversee, manage, and drive the program is considered to be a key element in the success of VHA's succession and workforce development efforts. (VA, 2007b, p. 14)

Several national VHA program offices located in the VHACO—the Employee Education System Office, the Workforce Management and Consulting Office and its HPDM Program Office and National Recruitment and Retention Office, and the National Center for Organizational Development—are variously responsible for VHA employee

---

[2] This section draws heavily on the *Department of Veterans Affairs Organizational Briefing Book* (VA, 2009b) and the *Veterans Health Administration Workforce Succession Strategic Plan* for 2007 and 2009 (VA, 2007b, 2009a). The material presented here was current as of spring 2009.

Figure 6.1
Veterans Health Administration Governance and Oversight

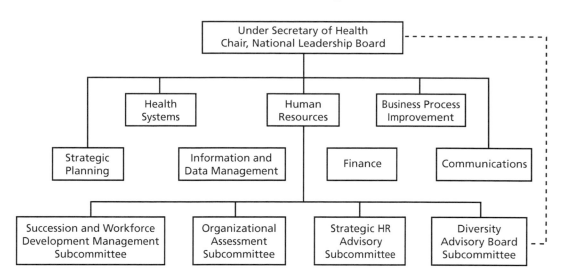

SOURCE: VA, 2007b, p. 14.
RAND *MG967-6.1*

learning (training, staff development, and continuing education needs), national work-force initiatives, program evaluation and assessment, and organizational assessment and feedback. They are overseen by and report to the Human Resources Committee of the VHA NLB and the relevant subcommittees. This structure is intended to ensure that the programs are aligned with and support the overall VHA mission, goals, and strategic plan and that field leaders and central administrators work collaboratively.

Recently, the VHA has been focusing on transforming itself into a learning organization.

In an article in the *Harvard Business Review*, Garvin, Edmondson, and Gino (2008, p. 110) define a learning organization as

> a place where employees excel at creating, acquiring, and transferring knowledge. There are three building blocks of such institutions: (1) a supportive learning environment, (2) concrete learning processes and practices, and (3) leadership behavior that reinforces learning.

The VHA obtained the assessment tool designed by the authors and is using it to survey its network and facility directors, to collect data on where it stands relative to other organizations and to understand where it needs to improve.[3]

---

[3]   The authors note that their online assessment tool aims to help "assess the depth of learning in your organization and its individual units. The power of the instrument lies in the comparisons it allows users to make—

As part of the effort to position itself as a "learning organization," the VHA implemented the Designated Learning Officer (DLO) Initiative, intended to provide a single point of contact (a DLO) for education and training at both the VISN and facility levels and to bring a systems perspective and integrated approach to the full employee life cycle. Each facility currently has a variety of staff who are involved in overseeing the education and training of different groups of employees. As one respondent noted,

> When you look at learning in that broader context, it is not your HR department, it is not your nursing education department, it is not just the library. . . . It's not any one of them, but it's all of them.

> We had asked that each hospital or health care system in VHA identify one person within that cadre to be . . . the voice or the focal point and provide at the facility level that systems approach to learning and workforce development at that medical center.

DLOs are not necessarily people with an education and training background. In fact, as another respondent mentioned,

> It was more important to make sure that they had the leadership skills, the change management skills to be able to help in the transformation of learning within our organization. . . . The technical skills of what education is were secondary.

An office in the VHA Employee Education System has been charged with developing the skills and competencies that these DLOs are likely to need to fulfill their learning leader roles:

> We're going to develop competency models for each of those three roles that I mentioned—the national, the VISN, and the facility—so that we can then use that model for skill-gap assessments, looking at the priorities of their training needs over time and then really just helping them be able to clarify their role and use it for hiring and performance management and succession planning.

In the meantime, the DLOs are participating in various activities (including national conferences for government and corporate learning leaders) to help them develop as learning leaders. They have also been asked to look closely at their own facility and start thinking about how best to use their local resources to move their facility forward as part of a learning organization. VHA leaders envision that one of the key

---

within and among an institution's functional areas, between organizations, and against established benchmarks" (Garvin, Edmondson, and Gino, 2008, p. 110).

roles that DLOs will play in the future will be in analysis and evaluation of the various educating and training programs.

Organizational Leader Expectations

As part of the overall transformation, a national VHA task force was chartered in 1996 to look at several issues related to succession planning.[4] As outlined in the 2009 strategic plan (VA, 2009a), the task force visited several national and international companies to learn about their employee and leadership development processes. This benchmarking resulted in the VHA's HPDM, which was adopted as the VHA's all-employee learning model in 1999.

The model is centered around eight core competencies and applicable to all four tiers or levels of employees.

The four tiers are as follows:

- *Level I:* frontline staff, those who do not supervise others
- *Level II:* work-unit leaders, those who lead the work of a natural group of people, either temporarily (process-improvement team leader) or as an ongoing role (foreman, section leader)
- *Level III:* midlevel managers (division, department, and service line managers), those in charge of a major function in an organization
- *Level IV:* executive leadership, those responsible for the overall functioning and outcomes of the organization (VA, 2008a).

The VHA's 2009 strategic plan describes the rationale for the model as follows:

The model increases access to training and development for the entire workforce, allowing VHA to move forward together rather than just developing a new breed of leaders at the top. The model increases the pool of potential executive leaders who come to the pool with a broader level of experience in both line and staff positions. Non-VHA applicants can be considered at all four tiers of the model. Because the model supports learning and developmental opportunities across the four tiers, there are enhanced opportunities for developmental experiences for employees earlier in their careers. The High Performance Development Model endorses the concepts of a "learning organization." (VA, 2009a, p. 70)

The eight core competencies of the HPDM are shown in the pyramid in Figure 6.2. The competencies follow a natural progression from more controlled accountability

---

[4]   This section borrows heavily from various undated brochures and pocket guides published by the VA.

Figure 6.2
The Eight Core Competencies of the HPDM

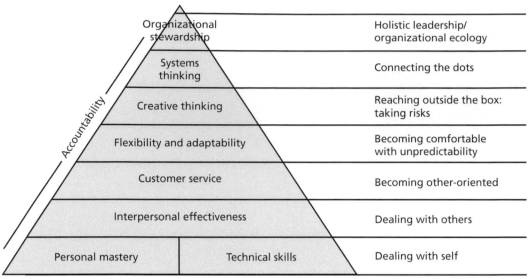

SOURCE: VA, undated.
RAND *MG967-6.2*

to more global accountability. As shown in the right of the figure, they also "form a natural progression toward interpersonal and organizational excellence" (VA, undated, p. 2).

The core competencies are defined as follows:

- *Personal mastery:* A lifelong personal responsibility for identifying life and career goals, being motivated to find out what it takes to achieve those goals, and continually pursuing them.
- *Technical skills:* The current knowledge and skills necessary to perform assigned duties correctly.
- *Interpersonal effectiveness:* The ability to work with, relate to, and communicate effectively with a variety of people in a way that is beneficial for all parties involved.
- *Customer service:* The ability to understand internal and external customers (i.e., coworkers and veterans) and to provide or exceed customer needs and expectations.
- *Flexibility and adaptability:* The ability and willingness to adapt to change in a positive, supportive manner even when differences of opinion or setbacks occur.
- *Creative thinking:* Willingness and ability to be open to different ways of accomplishing day-to-day tasks, offering solutions for change, and regularly evaluating whether there are new ways to improve processes.
- *Systems thinking:* An understanding of how one's roles and actions affect others and the entire VHA system.

- *Organizational stewardship:* Understanding and taking pride in how one's contributions and those of one's specific job responsibilities help achieve the overall goal and mission of the organization (VA, 2008a, pp. 5–7).

The core competencies are operationalized at various levels of the organization. The HPDM Program Office provides specific behavioral examples—by level—of how employees are expected to demonstrate that they have achieved a particular competency. Because our focus is primarily on the senior leaders, Table 6.1 presents examples of behaviors expected of Level IV employees with respect to each of the eight core competencies.

Table 6.1
HPDM Core Competencies and Behavioral Examples for Level IV Employees

Core Competency	Behavioral Examples
Personal mastery	Seeks continuous feedback about impact on others, through both formal and informal mechanisms
	Inspires and demonstrates a passion for excellence in every aspect of work
	Creates a climate in which continuous learning and self-development are valued
Technical skills	Uses technical or professional skills in creating new approaches to the field
	Nationally recognized as a consultant or adviser on current topics
	Fosters and rewards high standards for accuracy, safety, and constant improvement in all areas of the organization
Interpersonal effectiveness[a]	Conducts credible and prudent briefing sessions for Congress or the national media
	Exhibits clear, candid, and open communication in meetings, town halls, and other interactions; develops collaborative relationships across the network
	Breaks down barriers to effective communication
	Gives authority and responsibility to others
Customer service[a]	Shares resources throughout the facility in order to serve customers effectively and efficiently ("One VA")
	Bases strategic planning on customer feedback and projected needs
	Breaks down barriers that impede good service delivery
	Establishes a customer-oriented culture and promotes hiring of persons who fit that culture
Flexibility and adaptability	Responds to changing priorities and resources with optimism, encouraging staff to respond positively and proactively
	Stays abreast of and educates staff about changing conditions in the health care market
	Teaches the application of change-management principles

Table 6.1—Continued

Core Competency	Behavioral Examples
Creative thinking	Champions new ideas and approaches
	Encourages demonstration projects, pilots, and other experimental approaches
	Creates new functional processes that lead to the development of revenue streams or other gains in organizational outcomes
	Encourages and rewards risk-taking and entrepreneurial behavior
	Looks beyond the current reality to prepare the organization for alternative futures
Systems thinking[a]	Breaks down barriers and silos in the workplace in favor of high-performance work systems
	Understands the needs and complexities of the VISN health care delivery system components
	Shares the "big picture" with staff, including the consequences of not thinking holistically
	Recognizes and accepts global consequences of every decision
Organizational stewardship[a]	Demonstrates commitment to the network's business and strategic plans
	Encourages an atmosphere of trust and empowerment by example
	Provides a clear vision of the future and leads the organization through necessary changes
	Demonstrates commitment and accountability to the "One VA" concept
	Models behavior, attitudes, and actions expected of all staff

SOURCE: VA, 2008a.

NOTE: The examples in the table were current as of spring 2009 but may change as the VHA reexamines its leadership competency model and programs.

[a] These competencies were deemed "critical core competencies" in the performance assessments of Level IV employees in FY 2008, but they may change over time.

Approach to Leader Development

The HPDM is guided by several principles that undergird the VHA's approach to leader development.

These principles include the following (among others):

- Learning and leadership development are lifelong pursuits.
- All employees need to know how they learn best and be accountable for their own learning.
- The core competencies apply to all employees at all levels.
- The development of employees, particularly leadership skills, must be in concert with the strategic business goals of the organization.

- Rewards, recognition, and incentive systems are motivators for the continuous development of all employees.
- "Key contributors," who help achieve targeted outcomes but have no interest or aptitude for management, must be recognized, rewarded, and developed (VA, undated).

More recently, the model's goals have been updated to include the following:

- Expand employees' knowledge about business goals and processes and how they contribute to them.
- Create infrastructure for increased communication, both horizontal and vertical.
- Provide a variety of learning experiences, not just classroom training. ("Let employees into the kitchen rather than sending them to cooking school.")
- Place new emphasis on nontechnical competencies (soft skills, emotional intelligence).
- Use core competencies as common language and as expectations across service lines and facilities.
- Reinforce new behaviors and skills with appropriate rewards (VA, 2008a, p. 2).

To develop employees, the HPDM relies on six supervisory tools—often referred to as the six spokes of the wheel.

These tools are as follows:

- *Competency development:* Stages in an employee's professional life in which they expand their skills and knowledge to perform their assigned duties in an exceptional manner, whether it be through hands-on learning, classroom instruction, online instruction, or trial and error, for example. Competency development prepares them for leadership roles at all levels of the organization.
- *Continuous learning opportunities:* An ongoing learning process for all employees, occurring not only in the classroom or workshop but also while watching someone else perform a task, through trial and error, in open discussion with colleagues, through team analysis of successes and failures, and in many other nontraditional situations.
- *Coaching and mentoring:* Employees at all levels participate in a partnership to teach and learn from those around them, play a supportive role in encouraging and developing others, and participate in each employee's career potential and plans, sending a message that learning and growth are expected and supported.
- *Performance management:* Setting clear expectations, evaluating outcomes, and rewarding individual and team accomplishments.
- *Performance-based interviewing (PBI):* An employee selection process that focuses on demonstrated competency while defining the needed skills of the position.

PBI asks for personal examples of skills from the interviewee's past work and life experiences.

- *Continuous assessment:* A process that provides every employee with ongoing personal feedback about his or her performance and development, describing strengths and opportunities for growth while providing timely information to management on the level of competence and rate of development of the workforce (VA, 2008a, pp. 3–4).

In addition, employees are strongly encouraged and, at higher levels, required to have a personal development plan or individual development plan.

An individual development plan details career goals, skills and competencies, assessment content, developmental activities, and timelines. The plan should be based on a training needs analysis, career counseling, core competencies for the job or grade, and the HPDM.

Most of these development strategies are well represented in the literature and often identified as a set of best practices. As we discuss in the section "Selected Leader Development Programs," later in this chapter, the various ways of developing leaders are interwoven into the VHA's executive leader development programs, and the VHA strongly emphasizes coaching and mentoring, development or learning opportunities, and assessment and feedback. Coaching and mentoring are integral to each program because the VA believes that this instills organizational values and norms, creates a climate for learning, establishes trust and common goals, and translates setbacks into learning opportunities. Development activities can include formal classroom activities, informal observation, hands-on details or projects, and mentoring or coaching experience. Continuous assessment is also a key component and includes self-assessment through new learning technologies; 360-degree, 180-degree, or other assessments of core competencies;[5] and continuous feedback through coaching and mentoring.

How to Select

The selection process for executive leader development programs depends critically on PBI.

However, because readers may not be as familiar with PBI as with some of the other strategies, we provide a brief overview here.

Performance-Based Interviewing. PBI is variously referred to as competency-based or behavioral interviewing. The VA has a website dedicated to PBI that offers an introduction, guidance for both the interviewer and interviewee, and sample questions

---

[5] As noted earlier, 360-degree evaluation refers to feedback from those in the organization at the same level, above, and below the individual being evaluated (i.e., peers, supervisors, and subordinates), as well as external contacts. With 180-degree feedback, input is two-way, and the individual is evaluated by both his or her supervisor and team members.

linked to the HPDM core competencies that can be tailored to particular jobs. In addition, it also offers training in PBI. The website defines PBI as

> a method to increase the effectiveness of the interviewing process in selecting and promoting quality staff. With PBI, the interviewer carefully defines the skills needed for the job and structures the interview process to elicit behavioral examples of past performance. (VA, 2010)

According to the website, the rationale for PBI is that studies (not cited) have shown that the best predictor of future behavior is past behavior, so asking how job applicants behaved in particular situations in the past is a good indicator of how they would behave in similar circumstances in the future. The website offers a checklist for interviewers and emphasizes the need to review the important duties of the job and the knowledge, skills, abilities, and other characteristics required for someone to successfully perform the duties, generally through a job analysis. The next step is to plan a list of questions to ask all applicants; these questions should be tied to the job-related knowledge, skills, abilities, and other characteristics to avoid charges of invalid hiring practices. Table 6.2 provides some sample PBI questions tied to the HPDM core competencies for a Level IV employee.

Recommendations from supervisors and senior leaders are required as part of the application and selection process.

How to Develop
As mentioned earlier, the HPDM emphasizes leader development using multiple strategies, including coaching and mentoring, continuous assessment and feedback, and developmental assignments, among others.

Because selection and development strategies are closely interwoven in VHA programs, we use two selected leader development programs to illustrate the range of strategies used by the VHA. Both of these programs target high-potential executive leaders. Other VA and VHA leader development programs are described in Appendix G. Lower-level employees (such as those in the General Schedule [GS] 7–11 or 11–13 range) who are competitively selected as high-potential employees attend facility or VISN Leadership, Effectiveness, Accountability, Development (LEAD) programs. "High potential" is measured by three indicators—the desire to learn, work hard, and move into a leadership role; high performance in the current position; and evidence of the eight core HPDM competencies.

Table 6.2
Sample Performance-Based Interview Questions Linked to HPDM Core Competencies for Level IV Employees

Core Competency	Sample PBI Questions
Personal mastery	Tell me a specific time that you sought specific feedback on your performance from subordinates. Specifically, how did you use the feedback? Cite specific changes resulting from the feedback.
Technical skills	Compare what you know about the job you are interviewing for and your own knowledge and skill. What areas of development do you feel you will need to meet the job expectations?
Interpersonal effectiveness	Tell me about a meeting in which you had to tell others things they did not want to hear. How did you communicate those ideas to them? What was the result of that communication? If you could do it again, is there anything you would change in what you communicated or the way in which you communicated it? Why would you make those changes?
Customer service	In the past, how have you obtained and incorporated customer feedback into your organization's planning and service standards? Give specific examples.
Flexibility and adaptability	According to Peter Senge, the one simple thing a learning organization does well is to help people embrace change. Convince me/us that you are an effective change agent by describing an experience or experiences from your past.
Creative thinking	Describe a creative endeavor of which you can take ownership that had an impact on the efficiency or effectiveness of your organization.
Systems thinking	Tell me about a specific decision that you made within your organization that had unexpected consequences outside your organization. How did you deal with those consequences?
Organizational stewardship	Tell me specifically what you have done to create an atmosphere of trust and empowerment within your sphere of influence. What tangible results have you seen from your efforts?

SOURCE: VA, 2010.

These programs include a coaching or mentoring component, coursework, a personal development plan, and several opportunities for experiential learning through work on facility- or VISN-wide projects or task forces to provide leaders with systems-level thinking skills and expose them to the broader VHA. Thus, most of the high-potential senior managers and executives have already been through one or more leader development programs before being selected for those described here.

A key component of VHA leader development strategies is individual assessment and feedback, some of which is embedded in the leader development programs themselves, as we discuss later. However, other types of feedback are also provided, including 360-degree feedback and data from the VHA's All Employee Survey. We discuss these tools separately. We conclude this section by discussing the evaluation of leader development programs. The VHA is committed to evaluation and continuous assessment of its programs and considers it a critical element of its overall approach to leader development.

Selected Leader Development Programs. Here, we examine two VHA leader development programs in greater depth: the Executive Career Field Candidate Development Program (ECFCDP) and the VHA Mentor and Coach Certification Program.

Executive Career Field Candidate Development Program. The ECFCDP targets senior executives and senior managers (those holding positions one level down from senior executive) at the GS 13–15 level and other equivalent grades. To participate in this development program, candidates must submit an extensive written application and obtain the endorsement of their respective hospital director and VISN director or VHA chief officer. Beginning with the 2006 class, VISNs conduct PBIs and then forward applications that score average and above. A national rating panel, consisting of senior executives, scores the written applications and ranks applicants based on their total scores.

The ECFCDP consists of four six-month modules over a two-year period. A 2007 brochure titled "Developing Leaders at All Levels," published by the VHA, describes the program as follows:

> Successful applicants enter a two-year development program while keeping their current position. The first year includes three weeks of Health Care Leadership Institute, a series of audioconferences with Chief Officers in Central Office, and matching with a certified mentor who will assist in creating the Personal Development Plan. At the beginning of Year Two, participants, their mentors, and their local preceptor participate in a four-day intensive assessment center targeting critical skills for advancement. At this point, candidates select a specialized training experience to prepare for a position as Associate Director, Chief of Staff, Nurse Executive, or VISN/VACO [VA Central Office] healthcare program executive. Successful completion of the program does *not* guarantee a position but enhances the employee's ability to compete. (VA, 2007a, p. 3; emphasis in original)

We now expand on several components of the program:[6]

- The Health Care Leadership Institute is a key element of the program and is also offered separately to other senior executives. The course encompasses three week-long sessions scheduled over a period of six to nine months.[7]

---

[6] This material is drawn from an unpublished briefing by the VHA director of workforce development, "Introduction to the Executive Career Field Candidate Development Program (ECFCDP)," which the VHA made available to RAND.

[7] According to the 2007 brochure,

> Highlights include three assessment instruments with feedback and a 1:1 consultation with an executive coach; group coaching sessions with an experienced VHA leader; a two-day negotiation workshop; a media workshop; and key leadership books and articles. There is a strong focus on application of learning during the Institute and sharing outcomes with peers at the final session. (VA, 2007a, p. 4)

- Candidates are supported and overseen by a preceptor board, an assigned preceptor with whom they work on projects and details, and an assigned mentor. Preceptors, who are executive career field members,[8] are appointed by the candidate's facility or VISN director or chief officer. The preceptors review and provide feedback on the personal development program, support time and travel, and evaluate the candidate. Mentors, also executive career field members, go through a rigorous selection process that includes nominations from the VISN director or chief officer, submission of biographies and availability, and attainment of mentor certification. Mentors hold monthly telephone meetings and quarterly in-person visits with the mentored individual to discuss progress, concerns, and development. The preceptor board reviews and provides written feedback on the personal development plan; facilitates and reviews the 45-day experiential learning detail; facilitates, approves, and reviews the regional or national project undertaken by the candidate; obtains feedback from preceptors, mentors, and supervisors; and certifies that the candidate has successfully met the program requirements.
- Program requirements pertaining to projects and details are as follows:
  - Candidates serve as consultants on a VHA Systematic Ongoing Assessment and Review Strategy (SOARS) team. SOARS is an internal review initiative in which teams visit each facility every three years to interview staff, review procedures, and provide feedback to the facility to help it improve and maintain a culture of continuous readiness. The teams also highlight best practices that are then shared through the internal SOARS website.
  - Candidates are expected to work on a project in a leadership position that is either VISN-wide or national in scope. The project must be approved by the preceptor board that oversees all ECFCDP candidates, and the board receives final reports and evaluations.
  - Details consist of 45 consecutive days on a single facility's four- to five-member executive team or in a VISN or VHACO director role under an assigned preceptor, after which the candidate receives an evaluation and feedback. During this time, LEAD participants backfill positions in the candidate's facility as part of their growth and learning.
  - At the end of the first year, candidates, mentors, and preceptors participate in a weeklong assessment and feedback program at the VHA Assessment Center.

At the end of the two-year program, VISN preceptor boards determine whether the candidates have met all the requirements for certification. Candidates are either certified as having completed the program, allowed a six-month extension for further learning, or failed. The materials make it clear that the program does not guarantee

---

[8]   *Executive career field members* refers to executive-level staff: director, chief of staff, associate and assistant director, and associate director of patient care services (executive nurse). The ECFCDP is designed to train candidates for these roles.

placement in an executive position. Certification communicates that the candidate completed the training and development to the satisfaction of the preceptor board and the VISN director or chief officer.

Almost all the senior leaders with whom we spoke had participated in earlier versions of the ECFCDP or similar programs. Two mentioned that they had taken a yearlong detail at another facility during the second year. (This has been changed to a 45-day detail, as noted earlier.) One respondent also stated that an important aspect of the leader development programs offered at various levels (for example, the facility or VISN level) was helping employees understand whether they truly wanted to be in leadership positions:

> [ECFCDP is] the avenue towards directorship, associate director, chief of staff, and there are different tracks. . . . The whole idea is you are [not guaranteed an executive-level position] when you come out, except you've got general knowledge and, in some cases, specific [knowledge] if it happens to be a true technical field like government finance. . . . It allows you to become immersed in that and learn a little bit more about that. To me, one of the successes of a program like that is I remember that a young physician . . . within our network [leadership] program, who got into the program, went in thinking . . . that he was going to be a chief of staff, and when he finished, he thought, "I'm happy being a staff physician." . . . To determine that before actually getting into the battle is a good thing to know.

VHA Mentor and Coach Certification Program. The VHA established a national certification program for staff who would be serving as mentors, coaches, or preceptors in the organization's developmental programs. The goals of the VHA Mentor and Coach Certification Program include the following:

- to bring consistency and uniformity of content and experience to VHA mentor, coach, and preceptor training programs
- to enhance the quality of VHA mentors, coaches, and preceptors through experience and training
- to design and administer a certification process to officially evaluate and recognize the contributions of VHA mentors, coaches, and preceptors (VA, 2009a).

Training is provided at three progressive levels (resident-, fellow-, and master-level certification) that build on the knowledge and experience of each lower level. Certification at each level requires completion of both the training and practical experience. For example, certification as a resident mentor requires 25 hours of practical experience, while certification as a fellow requires 50 hours and master requires 100 hours.

An oversight body, the VHA Mentor Certification and Advisory Board, which is accountable to the Human Resources Committee of the NLB, oversees and administers the program. A national database was designed to assist VHA mentors, coaches, and preceptors in managing certification progress. The VHA Mentor Certification and Advisory Board began certifying mentors, coaches, and preceptors in FY 2007.

Feedback. Individual assessment and feedback underpin VHA leader development initiatives. However, other tools are also available, including 360-degree feedback and data from the VHA's All Employee Survey.

Individuals are offered the opportunity to participate in 360-degree feedback through the VHA National Center for Organizational Development (NCOD), which was established to measure and monitor the health of the organization.

NCOD staff meet with individuals to help interpret the results of the feedback process and to develop personal development plans that address problematic behaviors or weaknesses identified by the assessment. In our interviews, it was made very clear that such assessments are not used for evaluation but, rather, as a developmental tool.

An important part of the feedback consists of data drawn from the VHA All Employee Survey.

The NCOD conducts, analyzes, and interprets the All Employee Survey results and then provides customized feedback to networks and facilities.[9] The survey has a very high response rate—76 percent in 2007 and 73 percent in 2008. It has three components: (1) the Job Satisfaction Index, a 13-dimension scale that measures individual employee satisfaction with key job features; (2) the Organizational Assessment Inventory, a 20-dimension scale that measures employee perceptions of conditions in their immediate work group; and (3) a set of questions that measure employee perceptions of the general atmosphere, or culture, at their facility and map to four dimensions. The data are analyzed at the VISN, facility, and, where possible, work-group level. These analyses show longitudinal trends within the unit of analysis (for example, for a particular VISN or facility) and enable comparison with overall VHA averages, including statistical significance of the differences. NCOD staff prepare and present briefings to each VISN and facility and help interpret differences and trends. They advise the VISN or facility to focus on practical versus statistical significance (i.e., differences that are large enough to matter) and to give greater weight to patterns rather than one-of-a-kind findings.

---

[9] The NCOD has several other functions. For example, it conducts 360- and 180-degree assessments of individuals and is responsible for feedback and assessment of critical skills of executive career field candidates. It develops customized assessment instruments for network and facility leaders and conducts site visits to locations struggling with issues related to organizational health. It also offers interventions to improve organizational health. One such initiative is called Civility, Respect, and Engagement in the Workplace and was developed in-house. Respondents noted that this intervention had improved the culture and work relationships among the teams and facilities that adopted it.

Feedback is a critical element of the VHA's quality-improvement plan, which tracks and highlights trends and comparative standings. The findings are reported to senior leadership and taken seriously in performance evaluations. As one respondent noted,

> That feedback goes all the way to facility. Even then, you can break down to the unit level, depending on how well your mapping is done. We're able to get some feedback to supervisors as to how they're doing. . . . But the point of it is getting feedback from your employees and also demonstrating that you've done something with it.

Another respondent explained the process for providing feedback to staff:

> I meet quarterly with employees to give them updates on things, but predominately to hear from them—concerns, questions, suggestions. . . . We try to be very proactive about noting the issues that are raised and then taking action and feeding it back. And I have a workforce development coordinator who helps to organize the town hall meetings and to go with me and track things. And among the things that we do are feedback results of all employee surveys, and [we] hear from them things that we can do to improve the quality of the work environment.

Evaluation of Leader Development Programs. VHA program evaluation figures prominently in VHA literature and culture. The evaluation model in use measures four types of outcomes: reaction, learning, behavior, and results.

The 2007 VHA strategic plan emphasizes the centrality of continuous assessment, feedback, and redesign for all VHA leader development programs.

The plan states,

> Workforce succession program evaluation is a part of the annual strategic planning process and an integral part of the operation of each individual program. Programs are reviewed within the context of the overall workforce analyses and specific plans and needs identified by each VISN. Recommendations for program changes are then included in the update process for the national plan. VHA developed a general model for program evaluation and each program design incorporates the appropriate evaluation methodologies consistent with this overall evaluation model. (VA, 2007b, p. 14)

One respondent noted the change that had occurred in the VHA over the previous eight to ten years with respect to making such evaluations a central piece of every program:

The last five years we have been establishing a . . . stronger measurement function. . . . It's not just about making sure that we . . . "do evaluation" but . . . how are we driving and managing the data that we're collecting, and then using it to make better program decisions. . . . That's going to be our focus for 2009 moving forward and upgrading our systems and really taking a more strategic look at how we use the data for improvement.

The VHA uses the 1994 Kirkpatrick model for program evaluation with standardized data-collection instruments so that it can establish consistency across programs and track changes in programs' reported effectiveness over time (Kirkpatrick, 1994).[10] Some programs get higher-level evaluations; for example, evaluators will interview supervisors to determine the effect of the program on performance, jobs, and the organization in general. For a small portion of its programs, the VHA has begun to implement Level 5 evaluations (see Phillips, 1994) to, in the words of one respondent, "not just measure [satisfactory] learning but really look at the transference of learning into performance and actual practice on the job, and then linking that to business outcomes and return on investment." Because these evaluations tend to be very resource-intensive and may take longer to conduct, the VHA is careful about selecting the most appropriate programs for Level 5 evaluations.

Asked to give an example of program redesign based on program evaluation, one respondent mentioned that evaluations of the leader development programs, in particular, have resulted in changes both to program design and to the program components. For example, the evaluation showed less effect from the classroom, as opposed to the experiential learning through which participants were either getting one-on-one coaching and mentoring or were working on regional or national projects in an effort to apply what they had learned. As a result, over time, these programs have built in more mentoring, coaching, and experiential learning opportunities.

---

[10] Donald Kirkpatrick developed an evaluation model in the 1950s that, despite some criticism, is still widely used by the training community (see Kirkpatrick, 1959). It measures four kinds of outcomes that should result from an effective training program: reaction, learning, behavior, and results. Level 1 evaluation focuses on reactions, or how trainees feel about the training. This is the most common form of training evaluation and is typically conducted through posttraining surveys. Level 2 evaluation examines the learning that results from training, which may include both acquisition and retention of knowledge, skills, or attitudes. Measurement requires assessment of some sort and may involve determining gain scores through pre- and post-tests. Level 3 evaluation focuses on the extent to which learning is reflected in job-related behavior, or transfer of learning. Measurement of behavior is generally more challenging than measurement of reactions or learning; examples of measurement strategies include trainee self-reports, direct observations, 360-degree assessments, and analysis of artifacts related to the job. Level 4 evaluation is interested in outcomes, which are usually considered to be organization-level concerns. While sometimes focused on final, bottom-line outcomes, such as profits or revenue, Level 4 indicators can be anything of importance to the organization, such as customer satisfaction, employee turnover, or, in a health care context, improved patient outcomes.

How to Incentivize

Although we discuss the process by which individuals are evaluated in the sections titled "How to Incentivize," it should be noted that an important part of the evaluation process is to provide feedback to help employees improve. As such, some part of this discussion could also fit under "How to Develop." Respondents told us the VA/VHA is committed to performance measurement both for individuals and for programs.

The VHA tracks more than 100 performance measures in the areas of access, satisfaction, cost, and quality.

Deputy Under Secretary for Health for Operations and Management William Feeley, in a statement before the House Subcommittee on Oversight and Investigations, Committee on Veterans Affairs, noted that the VA's performance measurement system was a key part of the transformation of care that started in the 1990s. He explained the VA philosophy and approach as follows:

> Data on these measures are collected monthly and all performance is shared and distributed on a quarterly basis to the field facilities. . . . The aggregated quarterly data is also used to produce detailed annual reports shared with senior leadership and the field. . . .
>
> The successful use of the performance measurement system for driving quality is based upon widespread dissemination of information and feedback to individuals at all levels of the health care system. Also, it is important to link measures not only in performance evaluations but also incentives in a variety of local and national means. . . . I conduct individual performance reviews with each Network Director to personally review performance measure results for their VISN and to discuss plans for improving performance. (Feeley, 2007)

We now provide more details about the evaluation process.

Individuals are evaluated annually using a standardized online evaluation form. For each level, the form lists competencies along with several behavioral examples, and evaluators are asked to rate individuals on each behavior.

Individuals can be rated as "less than fully successful (little or no experience or needs practice or assistance)," "fully successful (competent, performs independently)," or "exceptional (competent, performs independently and is able to assess competency of others)." Evaluators must indicate how this rating was validated (for example, direct observation, patient survey, testing, or employee or customer feedback). If the rating is less than "fully successful," a training plan is developed, with follow-up within 30 days and a final rating once the training is completed.

The senior executives—network and facility directors as well as program officers in the VHACO—are offered performance bonuses.

For other managers and supervisors, there is centralized funding with ranges set for the different levels.

The next section outlines the key elements of the performance plan for network directors as an example.

Key Elements of the Executive Career Field Performance Plan for Network Directors. One respondent shared with us the Executive Career Field Performance Plan for FY 2008 for network directors (VA, 2008b). While the measures and the weights given to the elements change periodically, it is useful to review the FY 2008 plan. It consisted of the following five parts (weights assigned to each part are shown in parentheses):

- *Part A: Mission Critical Measures (critical element; 60 percent).* These performance measures include several quantitative and narrative measures. Around the mission-critical goal of delivering health care value, the measures are subdivided by domain of value—quality, access, satisfaction, business operations, and so on.
- *Part B: Transformational Measures (noncritical element; 10 percent).* Transformational measures are incremental measures designed to support long-term strategic goals, such as "Eliminate Health Care Associated Infection"; "Evolve a Comprehensive Patient-Centered Culture"; "Implement a Seamless Continuum of Follow-Up Care for At-Risk Populations"; and "Distinguish VHA as a Learning Organization," among others. The plan defines transformational measures as those that "establish incremental steps toward the Goal, reinforce corporate commitment, develop familiarity and buy-in, set internal benchmarks of progress and ensure the necessary technical, procedural and cultural adaptations to realize the Transformational Goal" (VA, 2008b, p. 7).
- *Part C: Financial Management and Business Practices (noncritical element; 15 percent).* Part C includes three sections: "Ethical Practices and Business Integrity," "Quality Control to Enhance Operational Oversight," and "Operational Efficiencies."[11]
- *Part D: HPDM Key Core Competencies (critical element; 10 percent).* The HPDM key core competencies are defined as systems thinking, organizational stewardship, service, and interpersonal effectiveness. At the end of the rating period, directors are asked to briefly describe personal actions or accomplishments that reflect significant achievement under these key core competencies.
- *Part E: HPDM Additional Core Competencies (noncritical element; 5 percent).* The additional core competencies are defined as technical competence, creative think-

---

[11] These categories represent specific leadership practices and strategies designed to optimize cost avoidance, manage workload to streamline flow and generate needed capacity, improve timely collection of debt, and reduce fee expenditure to a level consistent with health care market forces.

ing, flexibility and adaptability, and personal mastery. At the end of the rating period, directors are asked to briefly describe personal actions or accomplishments that reflect significant achievement under these additional core competencies.

One network director explained how the performance plan cascaded down to other leaders in the network and facility and how it actually worked in practice:

> We have a performance contract . . . between VA Central Office and the network directors. Then I [tell] medical centers [they] are now responsible for meeting this contract. So that becomes the medical center director's contract. Then the medical center director typically takes that contract and distributes that to the accountable person in the executive team and the accountable person in the facility for that particular goal. . . .

> Within the document, we also have an HPDM, the four competencies for managers and leaders, and we are asked to identify the demonstrations of achieving . . . each of those core competencies. [For example,] for interpersonal effectiveness, if I need to give two or three examples of how, as a network director, I am demonstrating my capability at a Level 4 of the HPDM. It is not a one-time situation. We monitor performance monthly.

Outcome

Respondents generally agreed that the programs and assessments were useful both for career development and in identifying high-potentials.

Overall, the small sample of network and facility directors who had been through these various leader development programs (albeit earlier versions) appreciated the programs and spoke highly of the overall support they received from the VA/VHA as they progressed in their careers.

One respondent noted that the VA's overall education and development program appeared to be unmatched in the private sector. The respondent had attended a leadership program run by the local hospital association to get a chance to meet private-sector counterparts who were members of the association:

> We would go around to different sites and learn more about each other. . . . I did a presentation on what VA had for education and development of their employees, and, frankly, we wowed them. There wasn't one of them that had that level or degree of educational offerings for employees at all levels—not just the senior executives, but all levels.

Another respondent eloquently described the attitudes and service mentality that these programs were attempting to instill in leaders:

> We work very hard here . . . to try to develop within our employees a sense of pride in who we treat and who we serve. You have health care as a worthy profession. But we have something more. That is that we have a mission and an opportunity to serve those that gave their yesterdays for our todays.

We also asked respondents whether they felt supported through their own careers and what more the VA/VHA could have done in this area. One respondent noted,

> They provide the training in specific areas periodically. We have a meeting with Mr. —, who is in charge of all the network directors, once every four or five months. . . . They don't do any overt training there, but they give us a basis to start looking from. . . . His big presentation this last time . . . was on variability. . . . Why do you have one network that has a readmission rate of 8 percent within 30 days and one network that has a readmission rate of 2 percent? . . . And that variability . . . needs to be analyzed and [we need to] find out what the issues are. And so, they're stimulating us all the time to think about things like that and to take advantage of the data.

Most of our respondents agreed that the performance appraisal system played a key role in identifying high-performers.

One respondent was somewhat more critical, particularly of the number of elements included in the performance plans, and believed that the plans needed to be streamlined:

> My performance plan is 20-some pages. . . . It's way too complex. It's way too cumbersome. When I'm doing the assessment on the people that report to me, I can . . . make them look really good or really bad depending on which components I emphasize.

Another respondent mentioned concerns about the performance appraisal system, its effects on cooperative efforts among the facilities, and the need to take stock:

> Some of the tools that are used to rank facilities are not especially well devised. . . . But they're used in a way that can have a disproportionate result on a person's assessment or a person's career. And it's one of the other less desirable aspects of the performance-driven system. . . . Early in this process, the incredible improvements that VA generated were a result of cooperation and working together and sharing best practices. And we do that in an amazing way. And I'm pleased to say that I haven't seen that eroded too much. But I do think that there is a risk of that happening in the future.

Other Comments on Improving Leader Development

Asked about selection for leader development, most of our respondents (regardless of background) felt that this should be open to all and that the question of whether senior leaders needed to be clinicians was a nonissue.

Here are some typical comments, including some from physicians:

I don't think the background of the individual in the position is really a germane issue, as long as they have the skill sets. Some of the best directors that I know, from my perspective, are nonphysicians. And some of the best are physicians. And likewise, there's some that are very bad that are not physicians and some that are very bad that are physicians. So I think it's more the skill sets that they bring to the position than it is what their training is, whether they're a physician or not.

The answer is that, well, it's not really a clinical entity. It's an organizational entity. Like running a surgical service or a medical service. . . . It's much bigger than that, because you're dealing with finance and contracts and facility management. So, a variety of people. If you have leadership skills well developed, and whether you're a doctor, whether you're a nonphysician, if you have those leadership skills, that will carry the day.

This is maybe heretical, and I may be struck down by a bolt of lightning, but I think that that argument is completely bogus. . . . I think being a physician in some respects gives you an advantage and a viewpoint that's very, very valuable to your leadership. And I treasure that experience. But I think it's a gross overstatement to say that you can't be an effective health care leader if you don't have a clinical background.

Some respondents noted that different leadership skills may be needed in different contexts; others mentioned the importance of having a strong team.

One respondent warned that circumstances in facilities or networks may call for different leadership skills (although there are some basic skills) and that it was important to look at the situational context:

There's some basic skills. I mean, you need to be able to manage a budget. You need to be able to manage people. In some situations, that means getting consensus. In some situations at other facilities, it may mean getting rid of people that are disruptive. But the basic skill sets of interpersonal effectiveness, creative thinking, systems thinking, things like that, they're pretty basic, but how they apply in any given situation is different. And there are subsets of those different skill sets that are important, depending on what the problems in a particular facility are.

Another respondent noted the importance of having a strong team:

I think that it's a function of leadership, training, and experience. And if you're an effective leader and you have the background and the training and the experience in health care, then you can be very good. But I don't think you can do it without having strong physician leadership and strong nursing leadership in your executive team. You've got to have a chief of staff who you support, who you trust, who will keep you out of trouble clinically and will do the right things. And similarly, for your nurse executive, you've got to have a strong nurse executive. And, hopefully, you have a very strong quality manager who can be a crosscheck on your clinical outcomes with your nursing and your medical staff. But I think if you have a strong team, then a physician can be an effective leader [as can a] nonphysician; a nurse can be an effective leader of a health care institution.

Asked what advice they would give to the military regarding leader development, three respondents mentioned that the duration of typical assignments was too short for commanders to be effective and that the military needed to rethink two-year assignments.

In fact, I think [being required to move every two years is] the number one disincentive for the military, in my opinion. I will tell you that in the time that I've been here, I've had probably a half-dozen different commanders over [at the Army base], all of whom have been very fine men and women. But the honeymoon is just barely over and they're gone.

I understand now that may work for active duty, but for health care, I personally think that they might want to think about maybe having a different set of requirements for the health services command, depending on what branch of service it is, because I just think it's terribly disruptive. I think it doesn't create a situation where you probably retain as many people. Certainly, it's difficult where you have a working spouse or significant other.

Back to the military, I just don't see [it] from the standpoint of being truly effective [in] 24 months, and during that time you've got to find a way to distinguish yourself and then move on. I just think that would be a very difficult environment for long-term gains is what I'm trying to say.

Two respondents offered suggestions regarding the development and sustainability of leader development programs.

Well, I guess the one piece of advice would be to . . . look at the best in class of leadership development and pick those skills that you as an organization believe best reflect what the mission of the organization is and create a training program that can be sustained, and also sustained in that each year it is going to be viable. How do you continue to improve that program so it is viable? Yeah. I think once a program's designed, it meets the need at that point in time; it does not meet the needs five years or ten years from now, and that has to be adapted.

I guess my suggestion would be to really focus on our developmental program and coaching, mentoring programs that we have, our structure that we've got, and the succession programs, like our succession committee and how that works. Because . . . you have to have some structure to it to make it work and to actually get support and buy-in and make sure things are working and assessment and everything. So, to really look at and focus on that.

Summary of Findings from Interviews

Table 6.3 summarizes the views of VHA leaders (as reflected in both our interviews and the materials provided by the VHA) with respect to the main categories of leader development. Once again, we remind the reader that this information was current as of spring 2009, and it may change as a result of the evaluation that the VHA is currently conducting.

Table 6.3
Overview of Themes Identified in Interviews with VHA Leaders

Area	Findings
Context and organizational environment	A decade-long revamping of VHA's management structure and approach to leader development
	Strong emphasis on leader development
	Focus on becoming a learning organization
Organizational leader expectations	Adoption of a structured competency model (HPDM) centered around eight core competencies applicable to all tiers of employees
	Competencies include personal mastery, technical skills, interpersonal effectiveness, customer service, flexibility and adaptability, creative thinking, systems thinking, and organizational stewardship
	Operationalized for different levels of employees through specific behavioral examples of how employees would be expected to demonstrate achievement of a particular competency
	Consensus that clinical skills are not a prerequisite for leadership (a "nonissue")

Approach to leader development	Several guiding principles including the following:
	    Leader development must be aligned with strategic business goals of organization
	    Employees are accountable for their own learning
	    Rewards and recognition are motivators for continuous development
	    A variety of learning experiences

	Six tools for development: competency development, continuous learning opportunities, coaching and mentoring, performance management, PBI, and continuous assessment
	Employees strongly encouraged to have a personal development plan

Table 6.3—Continued

Area	Findings

How to select:
    PBI
    Recommendations
	PBI a key component of selection process
	Endorsements from supervisors and other senior leaders

How to develop:
    Coaching and mentoring
    Workshops and courses
    Projects, including some at other facilities and positions
    Assessment and feedback
	Structured leader development programs that encompass several best-practice strategies:
	    At both facility and national levels
	    Emphasis on experiential learning
	    Trained/certified mentors and coaches
	Structured feedback from NCOD (data from All Employee Survey)
	Emphasis on program evaluation and improvement

How to incentivize:
    Performance appraisal system
    Promotion opportunities
    Performance bonuses
	Highly structured performance management system that tracks more than 100 performance measures
	Standardized online evaluation form that integrates the competencies from the HPDM (individuals rated on behaviors representing these competencies)
	Bonuses linked to performance

Outcome	Consensus that VHA system is good at selecting high-performers and at developing and supporting them

Chapter Seven presents our conclusions and recommendations for improving leader development in the MHS.

Conclusions and Recommendations

We were asked to examine the ways in which leaders (defined as individuals who are likely to be in command or executive positions in organizations) in the health care field are prepared and supported in the civilian and military sectors, to review the competencies necessary to be a leader in the current environment, and to recommend ways to improve how potential leaders are identified and developed for leadership positions in MHS.

We organized our findings around four topics that correspond to the four research questions underlying the study:

- desired attributes of leaders in the health care field
- military officers' perceptions of the current system of leader development
- lessons learned from civilian health care organizations and the VHA regarding leader development
- recommendations for improving leader development of health professions officers.

Desired Attributes of Health Care Leaders

To determine the kinds of knowledge, skills, and experience that organizations believe that leaders need, we reviewed a number of civilian health care leadership competency frameworks, the HPDM adopted by the VHA, and the military health care leadership competencies identified by the JMESP as necessary for successful command of an MTF or for other executive MHS positions. In addition, we asked respondents about the attributes that organizations looked for in their senior leaders—the skills, knowledge, attitudes, and experiences that organizations expected of their executives. Perhaps not surprisingly, there was remarkable consistency in the set of competencies identified both by the frameworks and the individuals who we interviewed.

The literature and our interviews converged on three common themes of effective leadership, regardless of sector or profession.

First, *management knowledge and experience* includes the skills and abilities to effectively manage financial, human, and information resources to ensure successful fulfillment of organizational goals. Respondents often described the need for both "hard" and "soft" skills. Identified common hard-skill competencies included HR management (such as recruitment, staffing, training, and evaluation and assessment), financial resource management (such as budgeting, asset management, and monitoring the use of financial resources), and information and technology management. The soft skills, or interpersonal and communication skills (with internal and external customers), were considered equally important. Some service respondents characterized these as "intangible" and "less didactic or technical" and included in this skill set being able to work on a team, building strong teams, mentoring and developing subordinates (e.g., acting like a "good parent," "empowering them to be able to do what they need to do"), creating positive climates that "people can grow in," listening to subordinates' concerns, inspiring and acknowledging contributions of others, and creating consensus.

Second, *leadership knowledge and experience* provides strategic and visionary guidance to help the organization meet future challenges. Competencies that fall into this category include visionary leadership (i.e., envisioning a future state and influencing movement toward it), change leadership (i.e., continuously seeking innovative approaches and welcoming changes as opportunities for improvement), flexibility and adaptability, and creative and strategic thinking and planning.

Third, *enterprise knowledge and experience* includes competencies that demonstrate sound understanding of the profession and the organization, such as organizational awareness or stewardship, an understanding of the larger context in which the organization operates (or systems-level thinking), and an understanding of the global environment. For instance, service respondents spoke about the importance of being "systems thinkers," understanding and operationalizing a strategic vision, being a "forward thinker" who proactively addresses issues, and understanding the whole organization and service-specific system, or possessing a "global perspective."

All our respondents stressed the importance of *educational achievement and competency in functional areas*. Several respondents also emphasized the importance of leaders who possess *strong values and moral character* ("a strong moral compass") in addition to knowledge, skills, and abilities. According to several civilian and VHA respondents, a strong values orientation (e.g., organizational stewardship, integrity, financial responsibility) is included in competency profiles for top executives.

Respondents were divided in terms of the extent to which health care leaders should possess and maintain clinical skills. Some physician respondents—both military and civilian—stated that the greatest credibility as a health care leader comes from being a physician. In keeping with this belief, the Air Force policy reserves command of medical centers and hospitals for physicians (MC). In contrast, the Army and the Navy have opened up these positions to all corps. Our military respondents referred to these diametrically opposed policies as "best in breed" rather than "best in show." Most respondents (including some Air Force leaders) regarded the Air Force policy as shortsighted and out of step with practice in the civilian world and places like the VHA, where hospital leaders were often not physicians. Several leaders noted that clinical skills do not automatically translate into leadership skills.

Military Officers' Perceptions of the Current System of Leader Development

Several respondents recognized the *complexity of the military environment and its effects on leader expectations.* Particularly among Army and Navy respondents, leaders noted that the military and their respective services had become quite complex on a number of levels: for example, the challenges of managing a workforce that now includes military, civilian, and contract workers; dealing with the stresses and demands of an extended war and the disruptions caused by deployments; and new productivity demands and attention to the "bottom line." All these are shaping what is expected of leaders, who is selected for leadership positions, and how they are evaluated.

Respondents in all three services identified *differences in opportunities for leadership and growth across the corps.* Several leaders in the Army and Navy believed that, when compared to MSC officers, MC officers are at a disadvantage in acquiring leadership skills. Some of these respondents believed that because of the length of time required for clinical training and the demand to keep these officers in clinical positions, it often takes longer and is more difficult for MC officers to gain the requisite skills, although they have greater opportunities to move into leadership positions. In the Army, several leaders reported that MSC officers received leadership experience earlier than MC officers. Other leaders pointed to particular corps that were perceived to have limited opportunities for advancement and growth—for example, NC in the Navy, SP in the Army, and BMC in the Air Force. As noted earlier, MTF command positions in the Air Force are limited to physicians.

Some Navy respondents criticized the Navy's "lock-step" requirement that an individual needed to be a director, then an XO, then a CO, pointing out that this overlooks other opportunities for individuals to develop and demonstrate leadership skills. Some respondents noted that rank does not equate to leadership and that physicians, in particular, were often placed in leadership positions because of rank without the requisite experience and training.

Although some respondents in all three services were aware of a set of formal leadership competencies endorsed by the military, most did not remember the name (JMESP), and few found them to be particularly meaningful or consequential. Across the services, few respondents mentioned these competencies without solicitation. Most respondents also characterized these competencies as something you "get" or "obtain," not demonstrate. According to other leaders in the Army and Navy, officers submit to the system or "fill in the blocks" to show they have "achieved" the competencies through a variety of experiences, but this reporting does not guarantee or even demonstrate that officers have mastered the competencies.

Respondents varied in their perceptions of how purposeful and systematic the services were in developing leaders. Most Air Force respondents considered the Air Force to have a reasonable and well-defined system in place for leader development and mentioned both the flight paths and development teams as the formal process for managing careers. Perceptions were more mixed in the other two services, with some saying the system did a reasonable job and others characterizing the approach as lacking planning and design, using words such as "happenstance," "serendipity," and "being in the right place at the right time."

How to Select

All services use formal and informal ways of selecting high-potentials, but perceptions about the efficacy of these methods varied. Most respondents in all three services viewed *formal evaluation reports* as one of the primary methods for identifying individuals with leadership potential, with below-the-zone promotions and "getting ranked" as important indicators of high leadership potential. Nevertheless, there was widespread concern about the limitations of these reports, including inflated ratings, subjectivity, use of "code words" as discriminators, lack of writing skills on the part of the raters, and raters being too far removed in rank from those being evaluated. Many respondents also mentioned the role of *command and selection boards* in identifying and selecting individuals for leadership and leader development, but some expressed concern about the "soundness" and objectivity of this process. A few leaders mentioned interviews as another formal and effective way to select leaders, but this did not seem to be widely used. Many leaders across the services noted that an *"informal system" of information gleaned from colleagues and word of mouth* greatly affected the identification of leaders and potential leaders and that these influences were often more important than formal methods in selecting leaders at the highest levels.

Some respondents, particularly those in the Navy, mentioned the need to *ensure that the pipeline of potential leaders reflected the diversity of the larger military as well as diversity of experiences, skills, and opinions.*

While a few were satisfied with the timing of selection for leadership opportunities and training, *several leaders in the Army and Navy argued that identification needed to occur earlier than it currently does.* For example, many Navy leaders believed that formal development opportunities often occurred too late in a career to be useful; that the Navy needed to be more proactive in providing opportunities to individuals before they were in leadership positions, rather than offering these opportunities "'after the fact,' when you take over one of these organizations." As discussed earlier, *in all three services, leaders mentioned that physicians did not receive leader development opportunities early enough in their careers and often lacked leadership and management skills and experience.*

How to Develop

Job Assignments. *Many leaders viewed on-the-job experience as the most valuable and effective means of developing leaders. However, not all respondents were satisfied with the emphasis on developing leaders through job assignments.* Some Navy respondents characterized the Navy's approach to leader development as development "by fire," in which individuals are thrown into leadership positions and unfairly expected to acquire the necessary skills on the job. Others felt that this was particularly challenging for physicians. Similarly, an Army leader believed that the Army could do a better job of giving potential leaders exposure to leadership experience so they are not experiencing the demands of the job for the first time when they take charge of an organization.

Most respondents agreed that diversity of job experiences and wide exposure to different types of jobs and responsibilities are important for leader development. Related to this, respondents from each of the services described a system by which individuals were given opportunities to experience increasing levels of responsibility and scopes of work, each role expanding their skills and knowledge as a leader (although more limited for specific corps, such as the MC). Several individuals identified not only jobs but also certain job experiences that equate to leader development opportunities, such as representing senior leaders at meetings; being placed in charge when leaders are on leave; taking on collateral duties, such as serving on or chairing a committee; and serving in staff positions or as fellows or interns. *Some respondents noted that the two-year duration of assignments can be disruptive and that longer-term assignments may help retention.*

Enterprise knowledge and experience were seen as increasingly important for military leaders as military operations become more "joint" and integrated (interservice, interagency, intergovernmental, and multinational). Across the services, *many leaders considered joint experiences to be beneficial to leader development; however, respondents did not tend to endorse mandatory requirements for joint experience and assignments, noting that the lack of joint billets made mandating them difficult.*

Education and Training. Almost everyone described receiving *formal education and training for certain positions and commands,* including Command and General Staff College and other executive leader courses. However, there were mixed views about the value of the current education and training offered by the services. Some believed that certain courses were valuable; others were more middle-of-the road, noting that coursework must be teamed with experiential learning. Leaders across the services cited a need for better writing skills and more instruction on the business aspects of medicine, particularly for clinicians.

All respondents described senior-level PME opportunities offered to leaders, including their service's war college and the National War College. *Almost all agreed that in-residence attendance at war college was far more valuable than completing the courses by correspondence.* War college by correspondence was considered something that "checked a box." However, several leaders noted barriers to participation, including the high opportunity costs of in-residence attendance imposed on both the individual and the service. Navy respondents were more critical of that service's war college in terms of the amount of time it took to complete the coursework, the limited number of slots available in these programs, the potential for doctors to lose their bonuses while they attended the courses, and the lack of planning in career assignments that prevented some from applying what they learned in subsequent positions. *Respondents were hesitant to endorse mandatory joint education, given the limited number of seats at schools offering JPME.*

Respondents across the services identified the value of educational and training opportunities provided by individuals and organizations outside of the military, many of which were sponsored by the services. These included graduate school, strategic leadership courses, and the Interagency Institute for Federal Health Care Executives. In other cases, leaders across the services described seeking out their own education outside of the military (such as those offered by the ACHE).

Mentoring. *There was widespread agreement across the services that mentoring was important for leader development*, and almost all respondents described personal experiences with mentoring or being mentored. Mentor relationships were initiated from both the top and the bottom. While some leaders noted that their service had a formal mentoring system, *almost all described informal mentoring and tended to believe that it was more effective than formal mentoring programs.*

How to Incentivize

Several respondents described how leaders were incentivized to participate in certain development opportunities because they greatly affected promotion and command opportunities (for example, the advanced PME courses). Other leaders related their own decision to seek education and assignments to promotion incentives. Several respondents mentioned that *retention was an important constraining factor in the ability to identify, grow, and mentor high-potentials.*

While the annual evaluations were regarded as important, most felt that they were inflated and somewhat subjective and, as such, did not provide good feedback.

Lessons Learned from the Civilian Health Care Organizations and Veterans Health Administration Regarding Leader Development

Our interviews with leaders in civilian health care organizations and the VHA mirrored other research findings about best practices in leader development, but they also provided some additional insights. Here, we highlight some practices that leaders in these organizations believed were important or effective.

An important theme that recurred in our interviews was the *importance of supporting leadership development at the highest level* and the belief that "leadership is as important as anything they can do." This includes investing in infrastructure resources and committing to managing the process of identifying potential leaders.

The second major theme that emerged from our interviews was the need to *develop a "living" competency model that is linked to organizational goals and strategic improvement plans and that drives the organization's approach to leader development*. In these organizations, leader competencies were infused throughout the leader development process—recruitment and selection, assessment of needs for professional and management development, development of programs, and evaluation. A good example is the HPDM adopted by the VHA, which stands on some bedrock principles and is inextricably woven into that organization's leader development programs and its succession planning and evaluation processes.

How to Select
As in their succession planning, organizations were very purposeful in their approach to the recruiting, interviewing, and hiring of executives and considered this an important strategy for ensuring strong leaders. Several executives reported using *behavioral interview questions* to identify individuals who possessed the competencies and behaviors they sought in their leaders, while others mentioned specific screening techniques to assess individuals' values. The VA uses PBI extensively as a selection and assessment tool. In addition to offering training in PBI, it has a website dedicated to PBI that offers guidance for both the interviewer and interviewee, as well as sample questions linked to the HPDM core competencies, which can be tailored to particular jobs.

Several respondents considered diversity issues when deciding whom to target. One organization felt strongly that it needed to be proactive to better ensure that the hospital staff reflected the community. Respondents from civilian organizations described diversity strategies aimed at ensuring that more women and minorities ended up in senior roles, and, in order to do so, they worked to develop them at less senior levels to create a pipeline. The VHA pays particular attention to diversity in its annual succession planning.

How to Develop
Respondents mentioned that their leader development programs went beyond the traditional classroom format to include some or all of the following: stretch assignments or details to leader positions, short-term projects overseen by preceptors, 360-degree or other rigorous types of assessment and feedback, mentoring and coaching, personal development plans, and structured reflection. An example of this is VHA's ECFCDP, a two-year program that incorporates almost all these elements. Some organizations also attempted to address gaps in the individual's development by providing targeted experiences and assignments. This approach differs from that of the military, in which officers tend to have a more rigid, prescribed institutional pattern of development as they progress through

their careers. Also, in contrast to the military, self-development activities were not cited as important. Next, we highlight some specific promising strategies.

Job Assignments. Many organizations assigned *short-term projects* (or, in a few cases, short-term rotations) as a means of exposing leaders and potential leaders to multiple facets of the organization and providing opportunities to try out new skills and apply new knowledge. The VHA, for example, builds 45-day details into its executive leader development programs to allow individuals to experience the full range of responsibilities in a higher-level position, away from their own facility. One civilian organization has a "top ten project list" based on the organization's strategic priorities, which they assign to top performers and directors or managers they "don't want to lose." Other individuals believed that development activities should expose leaders or potential leaders to different viewpoints and perspectives, suggesting that breadth of experience is a key attribute for senior executives.

Coaching and Mentoring. In one large system and in the VHA, *coaching was used mostly as a form of development.* Civilian respondents who had used coaches often described the arrangement as the most valuable development opportunity they encountered. Mentoring, which is generally an in-house activity, pairs a senior, experienced manager with a junior employee, although the employee may seek other mentors on his or her own. *Most civilian respondents felt that formal mentoring did not work as well as informal mentoring* because of the difficulty of "matching" interests and personalities. *In contrast, the VHA has invested considerable time and effort into training and certifying coaches and mentors and in assigning mentors and preceptors to individuals in higher-level leader development programs.* The VHA believes that coaching and mentoring instills organizational values and norms, creates a climate for learning, establishes trust and common goals, and translates setbacks into learning opportunities. To reinforce the importance of coaching and mentoring, the VHA weights such activities in evaluations of senior staff.

Cross-Functional and Team Development. Some civilian executives described the *need for cross-functional and customized approaches to professional development, including team leader development.* According to one executive, providing cross-functional or interdisciplinary opportunities helps cut across silos in the organizations. An excellent example is LENS, sponsored by the NCHL, which explicitly requires participating teams to include individuals from different areas of the organization and fosters information exchange across organizations in its leader development programs. One organization assigned administrator and physician pairs to attend its parent-company leader development program because it was viewed as a "best practice" among high-performing organizations.

360-Degree Feedback. This multisource feedback method is a way of systematically collecting perceptions of an individual's performance from different viewpoints, including peers, direct reports, supervisors, and stakeholders, such as customers and suppliers. *Both civilian organizations and the VHA were adamant about not making 360-*

degree feedback part of formal evaluations but instead using it to help individuals develop growth plans to address the various needs identified by these assessments.

Program Evaluation. *The VHA and several civilian health care organizations stressed the need to build in formal, rigorous evaluation as an integral component of the program design and development process.* VHA respondents stressed the importance of measuring the effect of all programs at several different levels (using, for example, Kirkpatrick's four-level model of program evaluation). For the handful of critical development programs, they recommended measuring the return on investment as well (Level 5) to ensure that these programs were meeting strategic goals effectively and efficiently.

How to Incentivize

Both civilian organizations in our sample and the VHA involved top executives in some form of annual performance-based evaluation. *These processes tended to emphasize evaluation based on measurable metrics,* which were tied to broader organizational goals as well as individual goals; the evaluations generally linked to incentive or compensation plans based on weighted formulas. Some organizations seemed to focus exclusively on outcomes and measurable objectives (e.g., relative value units that rank on a common scale the resources used to provide each service or improve patient satisfaction, safety, or quality). While most evaluation systems assessed what leaders accomplished over the year, *some also assessed how they accomplished their goals. The "how" tended to be guided by leadership competencies, described by some as the "nonmeasurables,"* such as how an individual develops others, handles HR issues, or demonstrates organizational stewardship, among other things.

A handful of respondents noted the *importance of nonpecuniary rewards and recognition for leaders and emerging leaders.* Such rewards could include providing those with demonstrated talent or accomplishments a special title and project. Echoing our military respondents, some civilian respondents noted that inviting individuals to participate in select professional development programs was a form of recognition in and of itself, signaling that the organization sees their potential and wants to invest in their future.

Discussion and Recommendations

Overall, the majority of our military respondents believed, with some caveats, that the services did a good job of preparing military health care leaders for executive positions in the MHS by using a multipronged approach that included job assignments, education and training, informal mentoring, and annual reviews. Their comments—along with those of our civilian and VHA respondents—suggest possible avenues for change and improvement. To distill lessons learned from the study about effective ways to develop leaders for executive positions, we returned to the MHS's stated goal—to prepare health care leaders to succeed in joint, performance-based environments—and its desire to adopt a new paradigm for changing the way "we think and act," in particular, to move toward jointly staffed facilities, performance-based management, and total force and team development. We then looked for recommendations that would help transform leader development to meet the MHS's strategic goals.

Leader Competencies

The link between the competencies discussed in this monograph and organizational performance is not clear, and several military respondents simply saw these competencies as "boxes to be checked" rather than skills to be demonstrated. As the Center for Naval Analyses pointed out, if the MHS wants to become a more performance-based and results-oriented organization, it "needs to better align its leadership behaviors with its strategy to create a foundational purpose for its JMESP. Without this central focus, [medical executive education] courses might become ends in themselves" (Brannman et al., 2007, p. 7). Further, each service has its own philosophy on how best to cultivate and track attainment of the JMESP skills through a variety of medical executive education programs and distance learning courses. We mirror Brannman et al.'s (2007) recommendation to standardize definitions, criteria, and output measures throughout the JMESP. This becomes even more important as the MHS seeks to become more uniform or joint.

Many respondents across sectors felt strongly that softer skills, such as communication, listening, personal influence, and inspiring others, are just as (if not more) important to successful leadership than harder skills, such as managing budgets. Military respondents felt that not enough attention was paid to these skills and that leader evaluation and development programs needed to place more weight on these areas.

Recommendations. Based on our review of the literature and the input of our interview respondents, we propose the following recommendations for the MHS with regard to leader competencies:

- Reexamine the JMESP competency model to ensure that it meets the MHS's strategic goals, and infuse the competencies throughout the leader development process.
- Emphasize the importance of soft skills along with the hard skills in selection and evaluation.

Approach to Leader Development

How to Select. Military officers expressed several concerns about the selection process. First, they perceived the selection process to be overly subjective and lacking in rigor because of inflated OERs. Second, some respondents believed that not enough attention was paid to diversity during the selection process ("people with different characteristics and attributes").[1] Third, the lock-step assignment system of leader development prevented some officers from demonstrating leadership potential through other means or assignments. Quality of performance should be emphasized in every assignment rather than only in selective assignments so that all high-potential individuals, even the "silent leaders," can have a chance to take advantage of leadership opportunities. Fourth, respondents criticized the Air Force policy of reserving command of medical centers and hospitals for the MC. The majority of our respondents—military, civilian, and VHA, some of whom were physicians—thought that this policy was shortsighted and that it limited without good rationale the pool from which commanders could be drawn. This policy differs from those of the Army and Navy and bucks trends in the civilian health care sector and the VHA networks and facilities, where the majority of hospital leaders are not physicians. However, some respondents also expressed concern about some of the corps being disadvantaged in competing for command positions because of structural barriers. If this is the case, it may require broadening opportunities and providing needed experiences to officers in these corps to allow high-potentials to emerge.

Recommendations. We propose the following recommendations with regard to the selection of potential leaders:

- Consider using PBI to recruit and evaluate officers for executive-level positions.
- Improve diversity among those selected for leader development opportunities.
- Implement a policy of "best in show" rather than "best in breed." In doing so, examine the health corps structure to ensure that all corps have equitable access to leadership opportunities.

How to Develop. All our respondents (especially civilian and VHA respondents) emphasized the usefulness and potential of assigning short-term projects, stretch assignments, or collateral duties to high-potentials in providing them with hands-on experiential learning and measuring their leadership potential.

Several military officers expressed concern that most physicians do not get leader development opportunities earlier in their careers and thus are relatively inexperienced in terms of command and lack management and business skills when they are placed in command positions at the O-6 level. Our respondents recognized that changing the system to provide clinical leaders with such opportunities earlier in their careers may be difficult and expensive, given the length of their training and the need to keep up physicians' clinical skills. Adoption of such a policy would require careful selection and early identification of high-potentials. It would also require greater emphasis on management and business skills in military education and training programs to address the perceived lack.

---

[1] This statement is based on DoD's definition of *diversity* as outlined in DoD Directive 1020.02 (2009). It is currently under review by the Military Leadership Diversity Commission.

Civilian and VHA respondents and some military respondents who were experienced with 360-degree feedback processes talked about the value of such feedback in clarifying strengths and weaknesses in senior leaders and high-potentials and helping them improve. All stressed, however, that this feedback process is a developmental tool and should not be part of a formal evaluation.

The civilian sector and VHA respondents emphasized the need for senior leaders to have a broader, enterprise perspective; organizations often encouraged participation in networks and outside courses that allowed for cross-pollination of ideas across sectors and organizations. Many military respondents also recognized the importance of external courses and joint education and experience but were concerned about the constraints on seats and billets. Most agreed that such education and experience should not be made mandatory for promotion. However, given the MHS's new paradigm for doing business, which clearly emphasizes "jointly staffed facilities" and "total force and team development," such education and experience are likely to become even more important.

While all respondents stressed the importance of informal mentoring, the VHA has made formal coaching and mentoring a centerpiece of its leader development approach. It has also set up formal programs to provide training and certification in coaching and mentoring. The military might find it useful to examine the VHA's approach; in the short term, it could recognize the importance of mentoring by giving weight to such activities in evaluations.

An important lesson that came out of the VHA case study was that program evaluation must be a central component of leader development programs so that the feedback can be used to improve and update the programs. This becomes particularly critical in a budget-constrained environment: Are leader development programs current and tailored to the military's goals, and do they offer a good return on investment?

Recommendations. We propose the following recommendations with regard to leader development in the MHS:

- Reexamine the overall approach to leader development to determine whether it is feasible to provide shorter-term projects or stretch assignments to high-potentials.
- Provide physicians with leader development opportunities along with business and management skills earlier in their careers.
- Encourage the use of 360-degree feedback, and make it an integrated part of leader development.
- Examine ways of providing and validating shorter-term and more tailored joint training and education opportunities for health professions officers.
- Recognize the importance of mentoring in evaluations, and consider providing formal training in mentoring and coaching.
- Evaluate leader development programs for currency and relevancy.

How to Incentivize. Some concerns surfaced regarding the formal evaluation process. First, our interviews made it clear that, unlike the VHA's HPDM, the JMESP competencies are not an integral part of the military's evaluation process. By congressional mandate, they are the established requirements for executive-level positions. As such, appropriate behaviors linked to these competencies need to be clearly disseminated, and officers need to be evaluated against these competencies and asked to demonstrate their mastery through appropriate behaviors. Second, many respondents were concerned about the perceived fairness of the evaluation system. For example, insufficient training in how to write such evaluations could disadvantage an individual in the promotion process; often, senior raters were too far removed from the officer to really know his or her strengths and weaknesses, and because most OERs were inflated, they did not provide a good assessment of the individual.

Some of our military and VHA respondents noted that a change in the length of typical assignments could act as an incentive to stay in the military. The two-year assignment policy may be disruptive and a disincentive to retention of really good people. Structurally, it may be difficult to accomplish, but the line community in the Army has been able to adopt three-year assignments. This implies better selection methods for high-potential officers because fewer will be selected for command.

Recommendations. We propose the following recommendations for the MHS with regard to incentives:

- Consider a separate evaluation process or form for health professions officers that integrates the competencies that the military considers important. At the same time, consider ways to reduce subjectivity and inflation in evaluations.
- Examine ways of implementing three-year assignments for health professions officers.

We recognize that many of these recommendations will require structural changes and may be difficult to implement. In addition, some may require difficult trade-offs. For example, selecting physicians for early leader development opportunities requires selecting fewer of them and necessarily narrowing the pipeline. This may result in overlooking some who have the potential to be effective leaders but may not have the opportunity to distinguish themselves early in their careers. Going to three-year assignments has the same potential downside. Emphasizing joint education and training may mean reducing emphasis on other necessary management or leadership skills and training. Nonetheless, the recommendations presented here are a useful starting point for discussion of how best to align leader development of health professions officers with MHS's vision for transformation.

Methodology Underlying the Sets of Rankings Used to Select the Sample of Nonprofit Hospitals in Phase I

This appendix provides additional details about how we chose the hospitals included in the Phase I sample selection process, as described in Chapter Two.

U.S. News and World Report Rankings

U.S. News and World Report ranks hospitals in 16 specialties, from cancer and heart disease to pediatrics and urology (see Comarow, 2007). Out of the 5,189 hospitals evaluated, just 176 scored high enough in 2006 in such measures of quality as mortality and patient volume to be ranked in any specialty.

In 11 of the 16 specialties, quantitative data largely determined a hospital's position. In the other five, as explained later, the rankings were based only on hospitals' reputations among specialist physicians. A hospital's initial eligibility in these data-driven specialties required meeting any of three standards: membership in the Council of Teaching Hospitals, affiliation with a medical school, or (to open the door to non-teaching hospitals) availability of at least nine of 18 key technologies, such as shaped-beam radiation and advanced cancer therapy. In 2006, fewer than a third of the hospitals qualified.

A hospital's overall performance is summed up by its U.S. News Score, made up of three equal parts: reputation, mortality, and a mix of care-related factors, such as nursing and patient services. The 50 hospitals in each specialty with the highest scores are listed. Hospitals on the "honor roll" (n = 14 in 2006) demonstrated exceptional breadth of excellence, with scores at least two standard deviations above the mean in six or more specialties.

- *Reputation:* For each specialty, a sampling of board-certified physicians was randomly selected from the American Medical Association's Masterfile of all 860,000 U.S. doctors (200 per specialty in 2006 and 2005, 150 in 2004). The doctors were mailed a survey form and asked to list the five hospitals that they felt were best in their specialty for difficult cases, without consideration of cost or location. The resulting number represents the percentage of responding physicians who named the hospital. For 2006, about 47 percent of the 3,200 doctors contacted responded to the survey.

- *Mortality:* This measure compares the number of Medicare patients with certain conditions who died in the hospital in 2002, 2003, and 2004 with the number of deaths expected after the severity of their condition is factored in. A score below 1.00 means that the outcome was better than expected; above 1.00, worse than expected. Severity adjustments were derived from 3M Health Information Systems software (All Patient Refined Diagnosis Related Group).
- *Other factors:* The final third of the score depends on such quality-of-care measures as nurse-to-patient ratios and the number of key technologies available. Most of the data came from the American Hospital Association's 2004 member survey; for the few ranked hospitals that did not respond to the survey, 2003 data were used instead.
- *Reputation specialties:* Ranking was by reputation only in ophthalmology, pediatrics, psychiatry, rehabilitation, and rheumatology, because mortality data are unavailable for pediatric facilities and are irrelevant or unreliable in the others. Ranked hospitals were named by at least 3 percent of the responding physicians.

Solucient Top 100 Hospitals

According to Thomson Reuters, its Top 100 Hospitals Program identifies benchmark practices by using objective statistical analyses of public data sources. The study focuses on short-term, acute care, nonfederal U.S. hospitals that treat a broad spectrum of patients (see Thomson Reuters, undated). At the time of our study, the program was called Solucient Top 100 Hospitals.

Solucient, now part of Thomson Reuters, uses data from public sources, including the Medicare Provider Analysis and Review data set and the Centers for Medicare and Medicaid Services Standard Analytical File outpatient data set, and Medicare cost report hospitals are classified into comparison groups according to the number of beds available and teaching status:

- major teaching hospitals
- teaching hospitals
- large community hospitals
- medium community hospitals
- small community hospitals.

Within these comparison groups, hospitals are then graded based on a set of weighted performance measures. Scoring is based on the following measures, which focus on clinical excellence, operating efficiency and financial health, and responsiveness to the community:

- risk-adjusted mortality index
- risk-adjusted complication index
- risk-adjusted patient safety index
- core measures score
- severity-adjusted average length of stay
- expense per adjusted discharge, adjusted for case mix and wages
- profitability (operating profit margin)
- cash-to-total-debt ratio
- growth in patient volume.

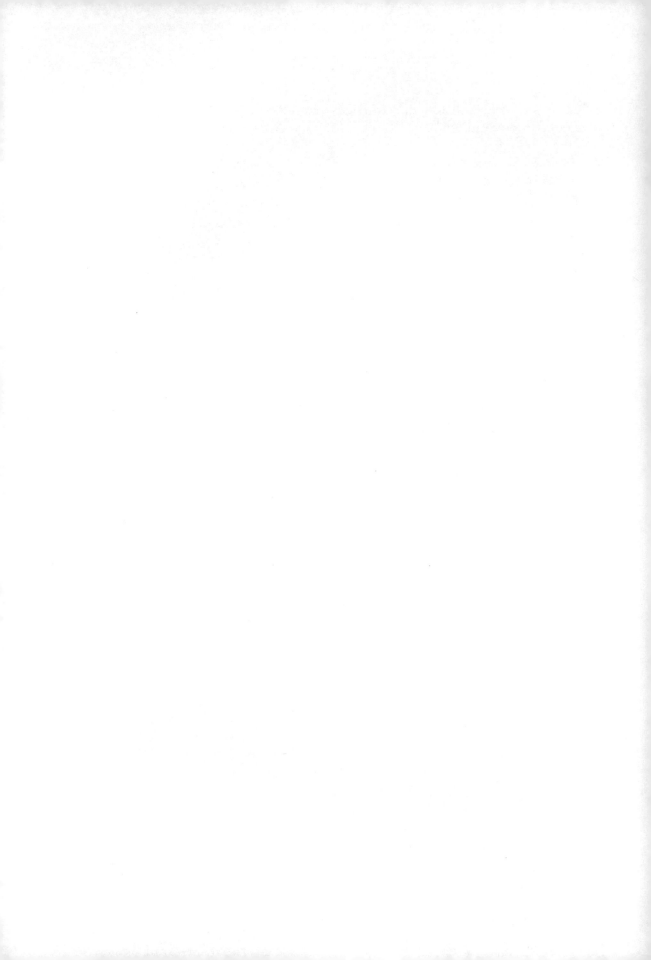

Development of Line and Medical Officers

This appendix offers additional details on the typical assignment and educational opportunities available to line and health professions officers. It supplements the information presented in Chapter Three. Our review shows that officers in most operational service components receive several common educational courses that develop their service-specific skills and knowledge base, commensurate with their rank and job-related needs (see Table B.1). The components also ensure that the officers serve in roles that provide increasing levels of responsibility and leadership skills. These officers are exposed to joint-level training early in their careers through service-specific education courses, joint individual training, or positions that expose them to joint environments. Most course curricula state that joint education in the early career setting is aimed only at "exposure" to joint matters.[1]

Table B.2 provides an example of the professional development of medical department officers, specifically military physicians' and nurses' career frameworks. We analyzed the MC and NC because they represent the largest corps in each service's medical departments and reflect the majority of personnel in those medical departments.

Our preliminary analysis shows some differences between the career paths of medical versus nonmedical officers. First, we found that some organizations in the medical departments of all services focus early career development on technical skills related to the specific profession (domain knowledge) prior to significantly developing military leadership skills and an enterprise perspective.

Second, medical department officers have more limited opportunities for joint professional education and training when compared to nonmedical officers. For example, some communities in the medical departments (specifically MC officers) are not required to complete PME and JPME I in the usual prescribed time frames, largely because of the need to complete medical education and training related to professional medical credentialing during the same period. Thus, the JPME I requirement is often deferred for medical officers until they are promoted to the rank of lieutenant colonel (see Headquarters, U.S. Department of the Army, 2007; AMEDD, undated, life-cycle

---

[1] DoD's Joint Qualification System Implementation Plan (2007) envisions a four-tier system of joint officer development, beginning at officer entry.

Table B.1
Professional Development of Nonmedical Military Officers

Professional Education Courses Common to All Services	Definitions and Descriptions	Career Time Frame	Examples of Positions Held	Examples of Joint Individual Training Opportunities	Joint Experience Potential[a]
Basic courses: Officer Basic Course, Air and Space Basic Course, Basic Community-Specific Department Officers Course	Focus is on tactical mission. Concentrates efforts on developing/reinforcing basic leadership skills, military knowledge, and other general military and common core subjects that apply to the specific community's mission. Joint awareness in the fundamentals of joint warfare and campaigning.	O-1/2	Platoon leader; crew commander. Duties include coordinating, supervising, and planning all operations for garrison, shore and ship, and tactical missions.	Community-specific schools that offer joint exposure, such as the Undergraduate Space and Missile Basic Course	No
Advanced courses: Captains' Career Course, Squadron Officer School, Advanced Community-Specific Department Officers Course	Focus is on tactical mission. Provides career-level professional education for captains to prepare them for command at company level and to serve as staff officers at battalion and brigade level. Joint awareness in the fundamentals of joint warfare and campaigning.	O-2(P)/3	Company commander; department head. Leads personnel to complete unit's mission, including all administrative and readiness tasks.	Attendance at Joint National Training Center exercise	Yes, but must serve in positions at O-4 and above to receive credit
JPME I: Intermediate Learning Education, Air Command and Staff College, College of Naval Command and Staff, Joint and Combined Warfighting School, Joint Advanced Warfighting School	Focus is on operational mission. Provides introduction to warfighting in the context of operational art and introduction to theater strategy and plans, national military strategy, and national security strategy. Develops analytical capabilities and creative thought. Provides education on joint doctrine development and joint strategic leader development.	O-4	Wing, brigade staff officer; joint task force staff officer. Duties vary by billet. Leads group of officers/enlisted personnel in creating plans, operations, and decision-support modules for missions.	Fellowship programs	More than 9,000 joint duty assignments offered to qualified officers; many available to officers at rank of O-4

Table B.1—Continued

Professional Education Courses Common to All Services	Definitions and Descriptions	Career Time Frame	Examples of Positions Held	Examples of Joint Individual Training Opportunities	Joint Experience Potential[a]
JPME II: Army War College Air War College College of Naval Warfare Industrial College of the Armed Forces National War College Joint and Combined Warfighting School Joint Advanced Warfighting School	Focus is on strategic mission. Provides education in national security strategy and guidance/command structures; national military strategy and organization; joint warfare/theater strategy and campaigning; joint planning systems and processes; integration of joint, interagency, and multinational capabilities; information operations and battlespace awareness; joint force requirements development; and joint strategic leader development. Total number of available seats for all services limited to 1,908.	O-5/6	Division staff officer; air, Office of the Chief of Naval Operations staff officer; commander; Joint Staff officer	Fellowship programs; business transformation conferences; joint warfighter conferences; attendance at resident JPME II institutions	More than 9,000 joint duty assignments offered to qualified officers; majority available to officers at rank of O-5/6. Prerequisite for promotion to general/flag officer
Capstone: Joint Functional Component Commander Courses Joint Flag Officer Warfighting Course	Focus is on strategic mission. Provides education in joint matters and national security, interagency processes, and multinational operations.	O-7/8/9	Joint task force commander; Joint Staff; combatant commands		

[a] Does not imply joint qualification or credit. A joint qualified officer has met all joint individual training, JPME I and II, and joint experience (of at least 36 months in a joint billet) requirements (U.S. Joint Chiefs of Staff, 2005, p. 8). The Chairman of the Joint Chiefs of Staff's vision is that the joint officer development plan will develop fully qualified joint colonels and captains (Navy rank) who meet all requirements prior to potential promotion to general officer/flag officer status.

Table B.2
Professional Development of Medical Component Military Officers

Professional Education Courses Common to All Services	Definitions and Descriptions	Career Time Frame	Examples of Positions Held	Examples of Joint Individual Training Opportunities	Joint Experience Potential
Basic courses: Officer Basic Course Air and Space Basic Course Basic Medical Department Officers Course	Focus is on tactical mission. To provide performance-oriented training to newly commissioned medical component officers covering basic soldiering/leader skills. Course provides basic skills and knowledge necessary to effectively function in medical units.	O-1/2	Nonleader position as staff nurse, physician, etc.; focus is on skill development and direct patient care. May have minor leadership roles but would not serve as a rater for subordinates.	Combat Casualty Care Course	No
Advanced courses: Captains' Career Course Squadron Medical Officer School Advanced Medical Department Officers Course	Focus is on tactical mission. Course is designed to enhance an officer's military frame of reference and to provide training in military medical service support operations with an overall working knowledge regarding the duties and responsibilities of medical component officers during periods of peace and hostilities.	O-2(P)/3	Nonleadership positions. Continue to develop technical skill sets and provide direct patient care. Most physicians enter residency training programs at this time. May serve in minor leadership role, such as education coordinator, but usually do not serve as rater to subordinates.	Medical management of chemical and biological casualties; logistic organization in theater of operations	Rare; deployment to sites such as Honduras on a greater than 6-month tour could receive joint credit
JPME I: Intermediate Learning Education Air Command and Staff College College of Naval Command and Staff	Focus is on operational mission. Provides introduction to warfighting in the context of operational art; introduction to theater strategy and plans and to military and national security strategies; develops analytical capabilities; joint doctrine development; and joint strategic leader development.	O-4/5	Key leadership roles begin at this level, including clinic officer in charge, brigade surgeon, head nurse, quality management director, and primary battalion or brigade staff. Many physicians enter Fellowship Training.	Executive Skills Course, Precommand courses; fellowship programs (nonmedical)	More than 9,000 positions on JDAL; however, limited number for medical personnel

Table B.2—Continued

Professional Education Courses Common to All Services	Definitions and Descriptions	Career Time Frame	Examples of Positions Held	Examples of Joint Individual Training Opportunities	Joint Experience Potential
JPME II: Army War College Air War College College of Naval Warfare Industrial College of the Army Forces National War College	Focus is on strategic mission. Provides education in national security strategy and command structures; national military strategy; joint warfare/theater strategy and campaigning; joint planning systems processes; integration of joint, interagency, and multinational capabilities; and joint strategic leader development. Total number of available seats for all services limited to 1,908. Very few offered to medical department officers.	O-5/6	Division surgeon, clinic chief, residency director; nursing division supervisor, assistant chief nurse, per Table of Organization and Equipment/Table of Distributions and Allowances. Also, medical department chief; director of medical education, deputy commander for clinical services, deputy director of nursing services.	Executive Skills Course, Commander Course; fellowship programs (nonmedical)	More than 9,000 positions on JDAL; current policy excludes most medical personnel from serving in JDAL positions
Capstone: Joint functional component commander courses PINNACLE curriculum	Focus is on strategic mission. Provides education on joint matters, national security, interagency processes, and multinational operations.	O-7/8/9	Corps chief, surgeon general staff; G-1 staff officer; Office of Under Secretary for Health Affairs Advisory staff.		

charts for physicians and nurses; and Air University, undated). In addition, the services' medical departments are offered very few seats at JPME II sites.

Third, medical department officers have few positions they can fill in joint organizations, and, as mentioned, DoD policy has been to exclude medical and legal officers from serving on the JDAL. Of the 9,000 JDAL assignments, most focus on operations or institutional needs; few require health services qualifications or focus specifically on the MHS.

Findings from Interviews with Army Health Professions Officers

The information in Appendixes C through E provided the input for the cross-case analysis reported in Chapter Four.

This appendix presents findings drawn from our interviews with Army officers. The analysis draws primarily on the 11 interviews we conducted in 2008, mainly with respondents who were MTF commanders. We also refer to material from our 2007 interviews, although they used a somewhat different protocol; not all were transcribed, and many were less comprehensive. We refer to all respondents in a gender-neutral way to ensure anonymity, but our sample included men and women. As a reminder, at the beginning of the interviews, respondents were informed that when we asked about leader competencies and development, we meant executive-level health professions officers, such as the commander of an MTF, chief medical officer, chief nurse, and others at that level.

Context, Organizational Environment, and Organizational Leader Expectations

Context and Organizational Environment

Many respondents (eight) described various structures that affected career growth for certain individuals in AMEDD or certain corps.

Most notably, several (six) commented on the designation of most command positions as branch-immaterial, and many believed that it was a fair policy because it allowed those with strong records to rise above others, regardless of the corps to which they belonged. However, one leader believed that certain corps officers were adversely affected by this policy. According to this leader, Army SP officers were often placed at a disadvantage when competing against other corps officers coming out of deputy command positions and so would benefit from having SP-coded field-grade billets.

> We need to compete across, but the problem with competing across is that the benchmark that people are competing [against is officers] coming out of deputy

command positions. . . . We don't have deputy command positions. The Medical Corps, the Nurse Corps, the Medical Service Corps have deputy command positions within the structure of the hospitals. The Dental Corps has their own command structure. Veterinary Corps has its own command structure. The SP has to play in lanes that are either open or that we force open. . . . And I'm coming from a perspective we should have them. Why don't we have them? Because we are AMEDD officers, and we should be afforded the opportunity just like the other five corps to be able to broaden our experience and grow the best officers, because we have some extremely fine officers that have been overlooked.

A few leaders reported that there are a limited number of O-5 command positions in the AMEDD, which makes it difficult for those seeking O-6 positions that generally require a previous O-5 assignment. Another noted that the MSC had eliminated some junior positions (e.g., deputy administrator), limiting career opportunities for these corps officers.

Related to this point, some leaders commented on differences in the opportunities for leadership growth and development across the corps, particularly the MC compared to the MSC.

Several respondents noted that MSC officers gained leadership experience faster than MC officers and that the majority of captain-level posts were filled by the MSC. Some also noted that without opportunities to command at the lower levels, clinicians were at a disadvantage. One identified a source of tension in deciding how to address this issue:

Medical Service Corps officers, on the other hand, have a lot more opportunity to command. Rarely do you have a Medical Corps officer who can command a company. Often, the first time that a Medical Corps officer can command is at a clinic level or, rarely, at a forward surgical team level. . . . I think that that's a disadvantage for the Medical Corps. . . . The first time I commanded anybody was when I commanded that first hospital, so I didn't get a chance to learn how to command and make those command decisions and who to work with at a command level until I was an O-6. I think that's a big shortfall, but how do you fix that? By taking physicians out of their clinical practice and putting them in command? I don't think there's a whole lot of junior physicians that are going to want to say, "Hey, I want to give up my ability to operate for two years so I can go be a company commander somewhere."

Another individual recounted the AMEDD's experiment with assigning MSC officers to command-line medical companies and believed that it was a positive move, noting that providing early leadership opportunities and acknowledging leadership potential early on was very important.

Some respondents recognized the complexity of the AMEDD environment and shifts that may be occurring.

A few leaders noted that the military, and AMEDD in particular, is a complex organization that includes multiple groups of individuals, including officers; reserve, enlisted, and civilian personnel; government civilians; and contractors. Others simply highlighted differences across the corps (discussed later). Some believed that the overall organization was doing a good job of integrating everyone. For example, one leader identified a "big cultural shift" that occurred in the 1990s, from an organization that was "stovepiped" to one that followed a more integrated "product-line concept":

> Medicine in the Army used to be very stovepiped; nurses go up their charge of command, just within the nurses, and the docs within the docs, and the [medical service] guys within the [medical service] branches, but there was no interaction per se on the chain of command and responsibilities, etc. . . . So we had Colonel Martinez, who later became two-star General Martinez, for the AMEDD and . . . he instituted a product-line concept [wherein] there were four product lines, like women's health, primary care, surgical and behavioral health, and you didn't have to be a doctor to be a head of a product line, and you could have been a nurse or an [medical service] officer. But the rating schemes, the OERs, were mixed, meaning that you had to have at least a noncorps in your rating scheme.

This leader went on to explain that while this situation caused an "uproar" initially, this structure now fits well in the organization: "I think AMEDD today is more immaterial in this way, especially when we went to immaterial commands, when before it was just MC's commanding. And I think that's the right way to go." However, another leader disagreed with this characterization and felt strongly that AMEDD remained very fragmented:

> So, I think what you find in many AMEDD senior organizations, you see a fragmented leadership style—it's stovepiped. You have nurses, you have doctors, you have medical service core officers, you have the enlisted, you have civilians, and it becomes difficult now for the leader who has not had that exposure and training to get them all on the same sheet of music. They don't speak their languages, and they have been so steeped in their own ideologies and idiosyncrasies, it's difficult to get out of that.

Others commented on the "turf issues" and "rivalry" that exist across the services. For some, this context pointed to the need for a unified medical command. As one leader explained,

The philosophies of the three services are so different without a truly unifying concept that we're working cross-purposes. So we end [with] . . . disagreements or protecting our turf rather than looking at the turf as belonging to all of us.

Another characterized the attitude among services as "us and them" and pointed to the fact that too many leaders view a joint assignment as a loss to the particular service. Similarly, another leader commented on the "rivalry" that exists across services:

A lot of people are afraid of what they don't know, what they don't understand. . . . There are no reasons that in my hospital, an Army hospital . . . where I'm short a psychiatrist, I'm short in primary care providers, guess what: I should have some Navy or Air Force physicians on my staff who can evaluate them fairly, and they can still move forward, and vice versa. We should be looking at those opportunities to integrate and make our folks comfortable around the other services. The mission is the same; we're doing things differently, but primarily it's very interchangeable. We don't do that, and again, that comes down to service rivalry and someone is afraid they won't get their piece of the pie.

Three respondents commented on how being at war affects leaders and leader development.

A few leaders reported that the wars have influenced expectations for leaders, who now need to know how to handle the effects of the "stresses of war" on those they supervise and on their families. Some felt that leaders needed to be more engaged and have a greater understanding of the stresses of multiple deployments on families. One commander explained,

The environment we're in now is an environment of, as you well know, sustained persistent conflict that affects not just leaders in the battlefield. It affects leaders here in the continental United States because we're caring for soldiers that come back. . . . [At some places] where soldiers are going out of the door on their fourth deployment or fourth rotation, . . . you have to deal with the stresses of the soldiers as they prepare to go, those that come back, and the family members.

Similarly, another leader believed that the persistent warfighting has changed the skills demanded of leaders, requiring them to be more engaged and empathetic:

I think today, because we're at war, it's more important that we be engaged and get down and talk to them [supervisees] about their families. . . . What I have found over the last two years and in this job is that engaged leadership makes a big difference. I send out emails periodically to tell them what's going on. . . . We've been in this war—what? . . . Five, almost six years now? So you have to look at it from what is the environment and what are the skill sets that we need.

Interestingly, one leader believed that the wars have had another effect, building stronger leaders who are "better equipped through their war experience than through some of the programs we have to send them to."

Retention and recruitment problems were seen as inhibiting leader development.

At least six respondents believed that poor retention was adversely affecting the AMEDD's ability to develop leaders. Some believed that it limited the availability of mentors for younger leaders. Others noted that losing quality individuals translated to a loss of future leaders. "There's a lot of people that have left the Army [who] would have been great leaders because the opportunities are different on the outside," said one respondent. Several identified contributing factors, such as the inability to offer financial incentives or higher salaries to compete with civilian organizations and to compensate for the length of deployments. One leader noted that the one area in which they are able to leverage some competitive advantage is "provider satisfaction" and workplace factors, such as the availability of electronic health records and ample support staff. Similarly, some also believed that family issues and concerns about lifestyle changes served as a significant barrier to leader recruitment and development. For example, one leader explained,

> A lot of people don't opt in [to leadership] because they think their lifestyle's going to dramatically change, and right now, they have control over their lifestyle. And, you know, when you're a commander leader and a chain of command leader, there's always somebody above you and there is a fear that, you know, my life is not going to be my own. That's why a lot of people don't opt in.

This leader and others also believed that many individuals did not want to attend the in-residence War College program because of the disruption to their families. For example, one respondent decided to forego the opportunity because it would have unfairly disrupted the respondent's child's high school experience.

A few individuals offered comments related to the length of time required for assignments and how lack of time in various ways affected leaders and leader development.

One leader believed that the two-year command inhibited leader development:

> Just commanding for two years is a challenge, because you don't get to know the organization for anywhere from three to four months. And then you really have only about a year to get stuff done, because then your replacement's already identified and your contacts and your replacement by change of command date. But the rest of the Army is going to three-year command, and we in the Army Medical Department haven't gone that way, and to be honest with you, I don't understand why, other than we're trying to get more people in the command. But the reason

really should be what's the best for the command, not what's best for the leader, and in my strong opinion, I think somebody who's in command for three years, with the leadership team there for three years, can get so much more done than two people in command over four years. So, I think we're shooting ourselves in the foot there. How do you get more people? Well, we've got to be able to identify them and put them into positions that are parallel to leadership positions and use them to the utmost of their ability. And I think we do that very, very well, but sometimes those people get burned out because they go from high-intensity job to high-intensity job to high-intensity job.

Another leader reported that leaders are too overwhelmed by day-to-day tasks to be strategic in their leadership: "I have a hard time doing strategic planning because I am so busy taking care of everyday work." One other respondent noted that decreasing hours in the residency program (a change that the respondent believed had occurred about ten years ago) did not leave enough time for leader development. This leader believed that a lot of important content, such as leader development, was squeezed out of the curriculum.

Leader Expectations

Many respondents (nine) believed that experience was an important criterion for leaders— particularly experience in a broad set of assignments, including operational and administrative experience.

Many stressed that leaders needed to be "well rounded," have a variety of assignments that gave them broad exposure to various jobs and settings, and demonstrate success in leading at these lower levels, as well as gain positions of increasing responsibility. One noted that some of this experience could be gained only from working in the military over time, which is why it was difficult to develop civilians who came into the military late. Four respondents believed that the breadth of experience should include experience in warfighting and that leaders should have a "worthy deployment history." Others stressed the importance of operational and administrative experience. (Management and business skills are discussed later in this appendix.)

Soft leadership skills were also seen as a necessity by many leaders (nine).

Many respondents considered "people skills" important for military medical leaders. To some, this meant being an "engaged" and "caring" leader who talks to staff about their family, rewards people, listens to concerns, acknowledges contributions, spends time with staff, and knows how to motivate and inspire others. Others emphasized the ability to lead and build teams and mentor others. As one commander explained,

I would expect the Army to place high value in those of us who are able to apply the soft skills across an organization, and be able to coach, teach, mentor, and motivate vastly different groups of people within our organization. . . . It is not enough to know the regs, know the rules, be able to write an operation order; that is simply not enough. You've got to be able to read people, interact with people, manage large groups of diverse people, and there are many leaders out there that are very ill equipped to handle that piece of the responsibility, much to the MHS's detriment.

Closely related to soft skills, some respondents (six) noted the value of communication skills and critical thinking.

These leaders talked about the importance of knowing how to communicate with others in a sensible way. For example, when asked what to look for in identifying potential leaders, one leader responded, "Bottom line: Can you communicate your thoughts effectively? Can you communicate that you're listening or at least send the message back that you're listening to each side of an issue? And are you fair?" Others stressed the value of being able to develop and communicate a mission, vision, and strategy.

Six respondents identified values or character as an important attribute of Army medical leaders.

Many of these individuals used similar words to explain the importance of being honest and open, living by Army values, and having strong character and humility. The following examples characterize comments we heard:

> The older I get the things that I value most become . . . the values. It's the honesty, it's the integrity, it's the ability to tell the whole truth. Those are extremely important to me. If I have somebody who functions well as a leader, at least the appearance is there, but [if] I can't trust them, then I don't want them to be a leader in my organization. So those value things play as big of a role as some of those other competency things because I don't think you can teach people the values, but you certainly can teach most people the specific skills they will need to be successful.

> [Interviewer: When you're looking for people that you would like to see promoted, or [who have] high potential, what are the qualities, the competencies, that you're looking for?] Character. First of all, character. And character boils down to a strong value system, consistent with Army values, first of all. . . . Someone decided to report that AMEDD's values should be Army's values: loyalty, duty, respect, selfless service, honor, integrity, personal courage.

Other respondents (six) believed that leaders needed skills and knowledge related to strategic or systems thinking.

These individuals described the importance of understanding and operationalizing a strategic vision, being a "forward thinker" who proactively addresses issues, and understanding the system and missions "two levels above." For example, one leader explained,

> It's very critical for a leader to look downrange or look to the future, where he wants the organization to go or be, and what kind of external influences as well as internal influences [there are] on the organization, the hospital, the unit, or whatever he's in charge of, per se. There are a lot of influences on the unit, and he has to kind of combine that with the goals, the objectives of his senior leadership, meaning, like in our particular case, the Surgeon General and the Chief of the Army. . . . We have to incorporate that in our long-term view as well.

A common attribute cited by many respondents (six) was that good leaders adapt well to changing conditions.

Many individuals used the words "adaptive," "adapts well," "adaptable," and "agility" when asked to identify what defines an ideal medical leader in the Army. Most believed that it was important for leaders to be able to adapt to changing conditions, particularly those that inevitably result from new positions and frequent moves.

Other respondents saw education and intellectual capability as important criteria for leaders.

Some cited the value of possessing a master's degree (for those without a medical or other professional degree), while others simply stated that education and intellectual capability were important. One described the "model" as "education, lead, education, lead"—meaning that individuals are expected to "hit the education wickets": Get a command opportunity, seek out more education, and so on.

Some respondents (five) felt that business and management skills and knowledge were important for today's MHS leaders.

These leaders stressed the importance of knowing how to manage an organization; understanding budgets, contracts, and metrics; and being facile with personnel and other administrative systems.

Many leaders agreed that maintaining clinical competency was necessary for credibility purposes and was often required for credentials and certain corps. However, many also acknowledged inherent challenges in maintaining this competency.

In many interviews, we asked respondents for their views on the clinical qualifications of leaders, the extent to which MTF commanders should be MC physicians, and whether clinicians need to maintain their proficiency once they have become executive leaders. Several believed that leaders did not necessarily have to be physicians. One was adamant that the private sector does not require executives to be physicians and disagreed strongly with the Air Force position on this. Another stated,

> I think a doctor, a nurse, or an administrator can effectively command a hospital. It's an immaterial job. You've got to know clinical, you've got to have a clinical understanding, you've got to have leadership, but you do have to [be] savvy on business practices.

In contrast, another leader believed that non-MC commanders were at a disadvantage (later qualified as a handicap but not a fatal one) and that they had a reputation of being "too far distanced from clinical medicine."

Many respondents (eight), with and without solicitation, mentioned that MHS leaders needed to have strong technical skills and expertise in their field in order to maintain credibility. One leader explained,

> You have to be clinically competent. I mean, that's just a given. You can't go up the leadership ladder because you couldn't do your job in cardiology or you couldn't do your job in surgery. I mean, . . . you can't have leaders that don't have their basic clinical competence or even beyond basic clinical competence, quite frankly, because they don't have that credibility factor with [those they will] be leading.

Several other clinical leaders attested to the value of continuing to see patients:

> I feel it's very important that you continue to have some patient care, because of several factors. One, it keeps your professional competency going. Two, it gives you credibility to the field, that you're still a physician, you're still seeing patients, you're still dealing with the same issues they are . . . and it really helps you be a better leader, too, because you experience those issues first hand.

> I see clinic one day a week, and I take calls one weekend a month, and I take the patients that I see in clinic and the patients that I get on the weekends off to the operating room. So I force myself to maintain my clinical activity. That is incredibly hard to do. . . . If I'm not upholding that same standard and I can't talk the same talk that they are, how can I possibly understand what I'm trying to make them do if I don't understand the systems that they're working with right now?

Some noted that retaining clinical skills was required by their corps (e.g., SP requires a minimum number of hours of clinical practice) or credentialing. Many, however, acknowledged the difficulty of maintaining clinical skills and seeing patients while also balancing other leadership responsibilities. One noted that it is often easier for certain specialties to retain clinical skills, such as a dermatologist compared to a surgeon. This same leader cited other ways to maintain clinical competence, including attending conferences, staying up to date with academic research, and participating in continuing medical education.

Although some respondents (five) recalled a formal set of competencies, few named JMESP.

Several individuals recalled seeing a set of executive skills or competencies, and a few remembered that there were around 40 (there are currently 39), but no one mentioned JMESP without further probing, and no one talked about these as being particularly meaningful. As one leader stated, "We have to kind of fill in the blocks of where we did what, what training did we take, what classes did we take to meet those certain criteria."

Most respondents attested to the value of leaders understanding how the other services operate and acknowledged that DoD is increasingly moving toward a more joint system. They were more mixed in their views about mandatory joint qualifications, however.

In most interviews, we asked respondents their opinions about the extent to which executive leaders needed joint experience and education and whether they believed that these requirements should be mandatory. At a minimum, all respondents seemed to endorse building better joint "awareness," but they differed in terms of how far they wanted to endorse requirements regarding joint education and assignments. Some leaders believed that it should be mandatory for high-level leaders (general, flag) to obtain joint experience and education. As one respondent explained, "I think it's critical. We are in a joint world. We need to speak joint language." Others used similar words, such as the need for leaders to "speak with one voice" and "learn their jargon and learn their systems." Another leader explained,

> We can't exist today without joint military knowledge, joint military training, understanding how Army, Navy, Air Force medical budgeting, funding, manning, staffing all work. We can't do it. . . . Understanding how the various services work and how to work all that stuff is absolutely critical.

While other leaders endorsed the idea of possessing joint knowledge, they were skeptical about mandatory requirements for obtaining joint education and training. Many noted that there were limited billets in which one could get joint experience and limited opportunities to attend JPME. Others were more critical of the content of JPME and its value for leaders. Still others did not believe that all leaders needed joint qualifications. For example, one believed that this knowledge was more valuable to warfighters than to leaders in health care settings. Another saw requiring joint requirements as leading to a loss of productivity. (Joint education and training are discussed in more detail later in this appendix.)

Other miscellaneous leader attributes mentioned included

- being proactive and able to deal with complexity
- giving others permission to take risks
- an ability to integrate military and civilian staff
- an ability to make decisions based on the good of the organization, not the individual.

Approach to Leader Development

Although our interview questions emphasized leader development—how and when individuals are identified for leader development opportunities and the specific opportunities provided—respondents often answered by describing who was selected as a leader and when. This likely had to do with how the services define leadership development: Much depends on experience (i.e., giving someone the opportunity to lead and gain on-the-job experience to develop them as a leader). As a result, the following themes blend both areas: identifying leaders and identifying individuals for leader development.

Overall, there was disagreement about the extent to which the Army is purposeful and proactive in identifying and developing leaders.

At one end of the spectrum, one leader strongly believed that the AMEDD had not done a good job of identifying and grooming high-potentials and that it relied too heavily on subjective means:

> You have to be willing to mentor and groom anyone, whatever their corps, whatever they look like, and just say, "This is a person I see with leadership potential, and I need to try and expose it and see where this goes." We have not done that in the Army Medical Department. Actually it's atrocious the way it does not happen. So now we have—and I have seen [it] too many times, this is not a rumour, this is first-hand experience. A physician will come to me at the grade of colonel, he's been a colonel two, three, four years, and say, "I want to be a commander, I want to be a general." . . . I have watched a couple of those officers that will say that to the right people, next thing you know, they're in command. Next thing you know, they're going to war college. They haven't had any experience . . . and it's wrong.

Another leader suggested that career progression in the Army is "based on timing and being at the right place at the right time." Still another noted that the Army did not have a systematic way of identifying high-potentials; either someone expresses an interest in leadership and command or a mentor asks him or her to take on a position. This leader also felt that "sometimes, we make an effort to grow everybody as that leader versus identifying the 10 or 20 percent to focus on, and that's a challenge as well." Still another leader believed that the AMEDD did not do a good job of identifying high-potentials. In particular, this respondent noted that AMEDD boards often opt not to use the "below-the-zone approach," and, as a result, many "super-achievers" are left with little direction. This leader stated that there is not a level of management that says, "You know what, this guy needs to be put in a key job and this is where you're going."

Other leaders perceived a greater sense of proactivity and purpose in the process of selecting and developing leaders. Many described the Army's overall approach as identifying potential leaders and giving them positions of leadership to "see how they do." Although some training may be offered, much of the development is expected to come from on-the-job experience. When asked how someone might be identified for the executive medicine track, one leader explained,

> It could be early on, as a major, and it could be like a general officer or myself, or somebody says, "Hey, this major has great potential. Let's try him out as a clinic commander or [in a] particular assignment and see how he does" type of thing. If he needs additional training at that level before he goes into that, we make sure that happens, but most of our executives are in the colonel ranks. But we have some in the lieutenant colonel [rank] and very few in the major ranks. But a lot of times, when people are identified as having strong potential, we keep track of them and see how they do, and then when they become a lieutenant colonel, there's two key jobs as a lieutenant colonel for executives that we put them in and that's a deputy commander or a division surgeon. So, based on how they do in those jobs kind of tells us how they're going to do as a leader as colonel.

Similarly, another leader cited personal experiences over the years that gave "the sense that people have sort of purposely [been] moving me into these positions: 'Let's see how he does with this, let's see how he does with that.'"

There was some disagreement about when leaders are and should be identified for leader development.

Some respondents were satisfied with the current timing, while several others believed that identification should occur earlier or, in at least one case, later than it currently does. For example, one physician leader felt strongly that some leadership development could occur as early as one's residency program:

> I would make the point that we have to begin intentionally training our CEOs when they're captains and majors. I think it's true in civilian [sectors] as well. . . . And by the way, I think we need to do this across the board. We need to do it in civilian medicine as well. So, I would make a strong pitch that . . . the place to

do it is residency, because they're young, they're impressionable, they're dreaming already of the kind of person that they want to be.

Others believed that leaders could be identified earlier, as majors, and be put into positions to see how they perform. In contrast, one leader felt that the Army identified people when they were too young and cut off opportunities for some. He noted that if one did not get into the Command and General Staff College, he or she would not be eligible for many subsequent opportunities and higher-level schools, which may cause the Army to overlook individuals with potential early on.

At least one respondent noted unfair differences across the corps: Some corps, such as the NC and MSC, tended to migrate individuals into leadership positions earlier in their careers compared to the MC. This leader urged greater "synchronization":

> So from a Medical Corps perspective, I think we need to focus a little more on after the doctor has done his residency and the first three to four years of payback time and [when he has] solidified his clinical skill sets, affording him the time to attend a four- or six-year-long course, like [a master of health administration] or whatever. I think that would do a lot to foster Medical Corps leaders.

Several respondents characterized the AMEDD's overall approach to development as one based on multiple means: assignments and on-the-job training, more formal training, and schooling.

As one leader reported,

> I think what's important [is] for us to . . . ensure that we get the officers into jobs that will develop their skill set and competencies, as well as get them the training and schooling that they need as well, to develop those competencies and then identify those who have excelled and those who have not excelled, in terms of how we can help them improve on their deficits, whatever it might be.

Another described a "model of education, lead, education, lead, education, lead, all throughout." Still another explained that competencies were developed partly through positions and partly through courses. Others, however, suggested that on-the-job experiences and placements were the most important form of development (see the section "How to Incentivize," later in this appendix).

How to Select

Formal Means. Respondents mentioned the importance of formal evaluation approaches, including OERs, 360-degree feedback, advisory and selection boards, and interviews.

Most respondents cited OERs as one of the main formal tools for selecting leaders (again, not necessarily individuals for leader development), but many were critical of the OER process.

Some leaders believed that OERs were a useful tool for "flagging" individuals to whom the Army should pay attention. These leaders believed that the reports gave a good indication of what supervisors felt about the individual's performance and their potential to take on more responsibility and accountability.

Although many observed improvement resulting from the "above-center-mass" system, many were still critical of the formal evaluations. For example, several respondents noted that the quality of the evaluations varies greatly depending on the rater and the quality of his or her writing. Several believed that these reports were often "inflated," although they acknowledged that the new system prevented "major inflation." One respondent said,

> We do have an inflated system. So I think it's true up and down our entire evaluation system. We're going to inflate. . . . You never comment on a person's negative attributes unless you think that person's going to be a detriment to the corps. You comment on their positive attributes, and sometimes you inflate those . . . for them to be competitive [because] everybody else is doing it. So it's hard to maintain honesty. When they put the "less than 50 percent rule in the top box" thing, I think that was very, very good because it forced people to do some segregation.

Another respondent similarly identified inflationary trends and pressures, noting that, especially in wartime, it is difficult to give officers negative evaluations:

> If someone is serving for me in a combat theater, I'll be hard-pressed not to say very good things about them, just the fact that they're wearing the uniform and willing to die for their country in a combat theater. And so there will be greater inflation through this war that will accelerate, I should say, the inflationary trends of an evaluation report.

Others believed that the reports gave "a very small slice of . . . that person's potential." One leader felt strongly that, without input from subordinates, the OERs provided incomplete information:

> It really is solely based on your superiors' opinions of you, which is formulated certainly by impressions that you leave with your peers, but only very rarely influenced at all by your subordinates. . . . Peers are often loathe to say something negative because they very much are in a glass house. So, if I say I have some real concerns about so-and-so to my commander and this person is a peer of mine, it would look, at least ostensibly, as though I'm just trying to bad-mouth them so I can get whatever it is they have. So I think the system unfortunately is set up so it's very difficult to know for sure who is the right person to push forward.

Another leader concurred:

We have a top-driven, commander-down-below rating system, and there's no peer input, and there's certainly no subordinate input. And you know as well as I do that there are people that look great to their superiors, and there are people who work for them [who] absolutely cannot stand them and would never work for them ever again if they ever had the opportunity to. . . . And so is that really a good leader, and is that a person you want to promote, because that person looks great to his bosses? . . . I don't think so.

Others raised concerns about who does the rating. One respondent complained that the senior rater is often too removed to make meaningful evaluations. The respondent also noted that some raters have far too many individuals to rate and believed that the Army line was doing a better job of limiting the number of officers for whom a senior rater is responsible. Another leader was critical of the new NC system that made the active and reserve components compete against each other. This leader believed that it was not fair for both to be in the same profile: A senior rater evaluates someone they see two weeks per year and someone they have knowledge of on a daily basis:

I don't think it's fair competition between the two groups, and, as you know, you can build a profile by having people who put in that profile who are center of mass. And how do you feel about putting somebody center of mass who you really haven't had that relationship with or [have known] well for a full year? Well, maybe not. So that person becomes your fodder for the active component folks who you have all the time, especially if they're both very good, but you see one all the time. . . . The much easier thing to do is to know the person better who you see and, you know, every week and you hear about every week rather than the person who you purposely make a phone call to once a month to see what they're doing in terms of their professional career and who only may drill two weeks during that year. . . . I just hope that we don't hurt our reserve component folks by doing that.

A few leaders reported developing strategies over the years to better utilize formal evaluation reports and detect "code words" and "discriminators" in the text. As one explained,

We've developed almost like code words. . . . On the OER, the senior rater will say "promote now" or "promote ahead of peers," and the senior rater will designate that the officer be selected for schoolings and positions that would normally go towards command. I think that's the code that has evolved—at least for clinicians. I don't know enough about Nursing Corps and Medical Service Corps.

Others reported checking in with "informal networks" and placing calls to validate official reports. According to one leader,

Sometimes the records tell you the truth, and sometimes they don't, but we use that quality check—or at least a check from somebody other than what we see on paper and our evaluations—to determine whether that's a good a fit or not. I mean, I've had a number of people that I've been called about who were recommended for some high-visibility leadership positions, and they will say, "What is your opinion? Do you think this is a good fit?" And, quite frankly, in a couple of cases I said, "I don't think so."

Some leaders (four) stated that they would like to see more of a 360-degree process integrated into formal evaluations.

Several respondents believed that incorporating the perspectives of subordinates, peers, and supervisors would greatly enhance the value of the Army's evaluation system and the quality of leadership. Some believed that the information would more accurately identify strengths and weaknesses and that the new system would create incentives for leaders to work harder on their relationships with subordinates and peers. As one leader explained,

If you've got a system where peers are supposed to be looking out for each other rather than competing against each other, with honest feedback from anonymous peers, you're going to get a lot more of an organizational ethos rather than an "it's me versus him for that next job" mentality. So it's a good system. Can we make it better? Absolutely. Can we do it easily? Yeah, we probably can. . . . We send out anonymous patient-satisfaction surveys. We can also send out the mid-tour, anonymous mid-tour, satisfaction surveys and grade your boss and grade your peers, just like we do with OERs. Imagine how much different people's leadership styles would be if they knew that they were being rated by the people that fell under them and their peers that they worked with.

Similarly, another respondent acknowledged that some individuals feared that using 360-degree evaluations would turn command positions into a "popularity contest" but still believed the benefits would outweigh the potential negative consequences. That respondent felt that obtaining anonymous input from staff at all levels would greatly enhance the quality of the available information about a leader's performance and potential. Still another respondent predicted that such a system could also help with retention and overall productivity because leaders would take more care in how they treated subordinates, and, as a result, these lower-level officers might like their jobs more, perform their jobs better, and subsequently stay.

Some respondents (four) reported that boards also played a role in selecting leaders for promotion, schools, and command.

Several respondents were fairly positive about the board process, noting that they did a "pretty good job of picking out people" for leader development opportunities. As one explained,

> I would say that the board process is extremely sound. That's the discriminator; that's the main discriminator. . . . The OERs are overinflated, . . . but I think the officers who sit on those boards, one, they know that, and then you're looking for other discriminators within that record. You're looking at the broadening opportunities they've had. You're looking at the field grade ranks, especially colonels, if they're in the war college or if they've graduated from the war college; advanced degrees, performance over time, are there similar words that are being said about this officer over time? And that's how they build that.

Of the four who commented on boards, only one was critical and urged that efforts be undertaken to remove the "good ol' boy" bias from the process.

A few leaders mentioned the Deputy Commander for Administration (DCA) Advisory Board as a "model" process for identifying potential leaders.

One respondent characterized this board as "a good way to identify folks who are strong leaders and have good skill sets to kind of step into these executive positions." That leader went on to describe the process and agreed with the interviewer when asked whether the process could be extended to include identification of individuals for development opportunities:

> It's run just like a promotion board. The officer's performance records are looked at and then basically . . . the goal is to fill a slate of vacancies that will come open in medical treatment facilities across the AMEDD during the next summer. And every officer is rated on a six-point scale, plus or minus, and then an order-of-merit list is finalized, based on how high a score [each officer receives from the] board. And then the officer, basically the number one officer on the order-of-merit list, you go to his first choice and there's a slating that you have to apply for when you apply for this board. And if you want to go to Fort Belvoir as your first choice and you're number one on the advisory board list, then you'll get slated for Fort Belvoir, unless there is some other . . . reason that would change that. . . . That is actually a very good idea of yours . . . to use those results to identify people who should go on for further professional development. Because that's a discriminating board, is what it is, and . . . you're evaluating for a selection for command, but those same folks are the ones that you'll look to groom [in] later years even if they aren't selected immediately. So, that's an excellent suggestion. . . . I don't see any reason why that couldn't be tagged onto that.

Two respondents mentioned interviews as another formal way to select leaders.

These two leaders stressed that interviews provided information that OERs and other written documentation could not, such as details about motivations and thought processes.

Informal Means. Personal references served as an informal means of identifying potential leaders.

According to five respondents, consultants and other leaders served as valuable informal sources for identifying potential leaders.

One leader described working with consultants to identify "less vocal" potential leaders. Others relied on key leaders to recognize "rising stars." When asked whether there was a system for identifying physicians with high potential, one respondent replied,

> Yes, and it's multifactorial; there's not just one system, and what we do is a couple of things. One is we rely, as well, on commanding generals and commanders and key leaders, like division surgeons or department chiefs, residency program directors, [graduate medical education] directors, to identify rising stars, what we call the "bench," that have potential to be future leaders or potentially they've done certain positions, to be a division surgeon or to be a deputy commander or to be a future commander. And they identify those and they let me know (or whoever's in my job), as well, and the consultants do, as well, within their populations. The 41 consultants we have—they look within their populations, too, and they identify those individuals.

Similarly, another respondent said that high-potentials were often brought to the attention of leadership via emails and calls:

> And so, you know, "You really need to look after Captain Smith because he is one who we need to groom to be a future leader ten to 15 years from now." We do see it, and [we also have] the officer evaluation report. But your question was good, because I think we run the risk, maybe, if there's too much inflation, of those officers who are high-performers being masked by all the others with the inflation. . . . You can't on paper differentiate that finally between the top 10 percent versus the top 50 percent.

There were mixed views about the relative value of informal versus formal methods of identifying potential leaders.

Some respondents believed that informal methods were superior to the formal methods, noting that official evaluations and documents were often inflated and not particularly informative. As mentioned earlier, one leader felt strongly that checking with "informal networks" and receiving information via telephone and email were essential for trying to identify the truth in official reports. Others similarly noted how difficult it was to truly recognize high-potentials based solely on written reports.

In contrast, others were critical of the informal methods—and to some extent the formal—because politics and personal connections often ultimately determined who received the leadership opportunities. For example, the leader who recommended the DCA Advisory Board process also noted that there had been occasions when some regional medical commands questioned the selection of the board and wanted their "protégés" in the position instead. Another respondent noted that there was a "political cut" to the process of selecting leaders for senior service college. Finally, one leader said that the composition of selection boards could affect the process:

> You can have a perfectly developed and executed leader development program, but when you're relying on a centralized board process to then select those officers and place them into commands, leadership positions, the outcome is strongly influenced by the board composition. . . . But I'm telling you that that is a factor that should be considered. . . . The results are sometimes skewed, depending on who sat on it. And one drastic example I could give you is, if somebody decided in the Army that, you know, for AMEDD boards, we're going to have just all line officers sit down and pick them. Then that would be a disadvantage to the position, the dentist, all the clinicians, because a line officer is more comfortable looking at Medical Service Corps records. They have similar career paths. . . . So, not consciously, necessarily, . . . but unconsciously, they would be skewed toward favoring the same striped officers, Medical Service Corps, versus the position.

Several respondents noted the challenges of looking beyond the "gunners," "go-getters," or "self-selected" to identify other officers with leadership potential.

According to these individuals, it is not always easy to look beyond the more assertive individuals to identify the less vocal ones with potential. One MC leader urged for improved efforts to identify the "silent leaders":

> If you look around, the people that get to be clinical leaders are the gunners. They're the people that . . . as a captain or a major [say], "I want to be [the] Surgeon General. I want to be chief of the Army Nurse Corps, is this personal goal," and they're clicking the boxes. . . . And so you've got a self-selected population of people who may or may not have the real true inner quality of a leader—the motivation skills, communication skills, people skills—but, boy, they can take tests, and they can go to school, and they can do all the metrics. . . . I think the first thing I would do is go out and try to find the . . . silent leaders out there that would love the opportunity to have some executive skills early on, and then the pool from which you could select your leaders would be much bigger. And rather than saying, okay,

he or she's got Command and General Staff College as a major, you know, he's got Senior Service College, as a lieutenant colonel. There are our leaders. I think there's a lot of people that could be leaders, but we don't offer them the opportunity. We don't go out and be proactive and say, "Is that what you'd like to do?" I think the Nurse Corps does much better than we do, much better.

How to Develop

Job Assignments and Experiences. Job assignments and on-the-job experience were described as important, but some respondents felt that the Army could do a better job of providing such experiences.

Many respondents described on-the-job experience as an important avenue for preparing leaders—whether it was taking on a new position or being given additional responsibilities as part of a current position.

Some leaders viewed on-the-job experience as the most valuable and effective means of developing leaders. One respondent commented,

> The courses lay a very marginal foundation for success. It's almost like a wide brush that gives you an idea of some of the things you may be exposed to. Nothing takes the place of getting your nose dirty, making a couple of mistakes, learning from the mistakes, getting you ready for becoming a leader down the road.

Others were more explicit about the ways in which job experience builds specific skills, such as learning how a budget works, how to hire and fire individuals, and so on. Others noted that on-the-job experience allows individuals to interact with individuals across the organization and across corps, which enhances their knowledge about what everyone does and their ability to communicate and lead. ("If you're going to be effective, get out there and talk to them.")

Several individuals identified not only jobs but also certain job experiences that equate to leader development opportunities. For example, one respondent regularly urged other leaders to "prepare their bench" by allowing high-potentials to represent them at meetings or by putting them in charge when the leaders were on leave. The respondent had learned to lead this way and explained, "That's the way you learn." Another leader provided several examples of being given opportunities to lead by serving on committees and described how these opportunities helped develop new knowledge and skills:

> [A leader] directed a zero-based budget review of the entire hospital budget and he assigned a team of five people to do it, and I don't know exactly who decided to put me on that team, but I was the physician representative to that team. We went first through a line-by-line budget of every aspect of the budget and every personnel position. It took 15 months of going line by line. . . . The best thing was the exercise

for me, because I know what zero-based budgeting is now; I understand a little bit more. So it was clear to me that that was intentional. . . . He wanted the job done, but he picked somebody I think that he thought would benefit from it. And then the same thing: He decided he wanted someone to chair the performance-improvement council that had traditionally been chaired by the general, and somehow it ended up being me.

Finally, another respondent believed that the Army could do a better job of giving potential leaders exposure to leadership experience so they are not experiencing the demands of the job for the first time when they take charge of an organization: "Offer them pieces of those positions or [give] them an opportunity to sit in those positions for periods of time to have that exposure, so that when they're there the first time, it isn't when they're in charge." Within this group, some also argued that diversity of experience was important for leader development. For example, one respondent said that it was important for individuals to continually go back and forth between MTF and units in the operational force to acquire deployment experience. Another leader described the need to be a "well-rounded leader," which included a diversity of experience and "wide exposure" to different types of jobs and responsibilities.

While most agreed that giving people a range of experiences in different types of jobs and environments was important, at least one person noted that the Army was recognizing the value of allowing leaders to stay within environments in which they have experience:

> The philosophy in the past was, one, it's always the needs of the service. That's clear. Needs of the service is first. Secondly, it wasn't good to stay in a place too long. It wasn't good to command in the organization you served in. And then, before General [Peter] Schoomaker departed as Chief of Staff of the Army, one of the mandates was to try to match officers up with—if they're selected for a higher-level command—commands either they served in or command types they have experience in. Because they've learned the lesson that . . . if you've grown and you've had experience at something, you're probably going to be more successful than [if they try] to move you around.

Some leaders (three) spoke about "developmental" or "growing" jobs or positions as good preparation for leadership positions.

One respondent noted that much of the focus in the MSC was on how to be a commander: "So, you go through the normal jobs like the company command, executive officer, chief of a department. Those are the developmental positions and [you start] out as a lieutenant as a platoon leader in a field unit." Another leader recalled expressing a wish early on to eventually become a DCA and being told by the branch that the next position would be an XO job because "that is a good developmental job for a DCA." Similarly, one respondent explained that there were many opportunities for physicians to step up and take on leadership roles, such as service chief, department chief, head of a joint commission, or positions on committees. That respondent noted that leaders needed "to step forward and take on these leadership roles, and those are the growing jobs."

There were mixed views about the value of joint assignments.

Some respondents strongly endorsed the need for joint assignments. Several cited the value of operating with other services and learning to "speak a joint language." When asked whether joint assignments were important for medical leaders, one leader responded,

> They're very important now, I think, because I think we're going to be moving towards some sort of a joint medical endeavour. . . . We need to have more officers that are working in that environment. . . . But, again, a lot of people are afraid of what they don't know, what they don't understand, so we need to get officers at a more junior level out there. . . . We should be looking at those opportunities to integrate and make our folks comfortable around the other services. The mission is the same. We're doing things differently, but primarily it's very interchangeable. We don't do that, and again, that comes down to service rivalry and someone is afraid they won't get their piece of the pie.

Similarly, another leader noted,

> I do believe . . . that is it important for officers to get joint experience through assignments—certainly at the field grade and possibly even company grade—but certainly as they're going through their career and getting to be field-grade rank. And why? Because the Department of Defense in general is going in that direction. The provision of medical care, combat health support, or peacetime health support lends itself to "jointness" as much if not more than any other functional area the Department of Defense has. . . . Certainly, at our combat support hospitals (so corps level and above) and back here in the states, the delivered health care can easily be delivered with the same quality or the same standards across the services and intermingling those assets as need be. So, we're seeing that in the hospitals.

This leader went on to argue for an expanded definition of *joint* and opportunities to develop joint skills and knowledge through assignments, preferably early in one's career:

> There are assigned opportunities now, depending on how you define *jointness* in inner agencies, across the services, and with coalition partners. And so the expanded definition of what I'd like to use for *joint*: There are a number of opportunities. If we had an officer . . . that we had failed . . . to properly career develop in the vein of jointness and they made the rank of colonel, . . . it's not a problem. We can get

an adjoined credit, that joint experience for them as a colonel. . . . You're right, joint qualification system is in play. It's very important to the Army. I believe it should be important, and it is, and we should formalize that within the AMEDD.

Yet another leader cited personal experience in a joint billet and the value of working for the TRICARE Management Agency with the other 12 regions. The respondent described it as a "great professional education experience," adding, "You learn from watching how each of the services approaches the delivery of health care."

Others were a bit more skeptical about the value of joint assignments. Some noted that there were not enough billets for leaders to serve in joint assignments. Others believed that not all jobs required joint assignments. Still others were concerned about the consequences of moving more medical leaders into joint assignments. One believed that it would lead to a loss of productivity. Another thought that it would interfere with the mission of providing warrior care. Yet another noted that the AMEDD would need to grow in size to offset the loss of positions.

Education and Training. Respondents noted several reservations about the current mix of training and education offered to medical leaders in the Army.

In general, there were mixed views about the current education and training offered by the Army and AMEDD in particular.

Some were proponents of various offerings and believed that certain courses were valuable. Others were more middle-of-the road, noting that the courses and training provided exposure to important information, but that true learning comes from on-the-job experiences (as discussed earlier). For example, one leader noted that the executive leader courses touched on topics "very lightly" and that, in general, they provided a "very marginal foundation for success." Similarly, another leader reported that formal centralized education provided some useful training on "how to command" and some exposure to budget and finance issues, but that "really you've got to get out there and do that to learn all that stuff."

Finally, a few were quite critical of specific offerings. One respondent believed that the Command and General Staff College was a "waste of time" and felt strongly that it should be tailored more to AMEDD personnel and specific corps. Another leader reported that the executive skills training program was weak: "They don't have the relevant experience to talk to you about what you need to do." Still another was extremely disappointed with correspondence courses, citing difficulty recalling "a single thing learned" in advanced courses taken online.

Some leaders valued the senior service colleges and the Army War College, but several noted barriers to participation.

One leader described senior service colleges as the single best preparation for a command position. Others noted that they learned a lot from attending the Army War College (e.g., strategic thinking, "how to think outside just the Army box") and believed that more seats were needed. Several strongly favored the residence option over the distance program but recognized the difficulty of participating in that option. One leader noted that doing the program online does not offer the valuable opportunity to network and interact with other officers. Another described the distance learning program as "painful." Several acknowledged that participating in the residence option was difficult if one has a family. For example, one leader had to forgo the opportunity in order to avoid disrupting their child's education.

Similar to comments about joint assignments, several leaders expressed a need for new joint education opportunities. For example, one respondent believed that joint education could be integrated into the captain's career course and other ILE, arguing that JPME could be distilled to a three- to four-month joint course for medical professionals. Another simply noted that "the curriculum of the course can't be so onerous that the doctors won't sign up to play."

A few respondents (three) noted the value of courses and education that provide exposure to the practices and ideas of organizations outside of the military, such as the civilian health care industry.

One leader recalled a valuable strategic leadership course offered by the Army that brought in industry leaders:

> I learned so much. And he brought in CEOs from other companies and we had a chance to interact with them to tell them how we do business, and we were able to learn about how they execute as CEOs. And I thought that was very effective in terms of looking outside the military. Sometime, we get really stuck in our own world. So I would recommend that they not be so boxed in to just what the military leaders say, but do some research, and interview others who have been there and done it.

Others believed that the Army needed to partner with industry to provide better educational opportunities for leaders, such as internships and fellowships that expose individuals to settings outside of the military.

Several leaders shared specific criticisms and recommendations for how to improve education and training.

In terms of course content, several respondents cited a need for more instruction on the business aspects of medicine, such as finance and budget, particularly for clinicians. For example, one leader said that the Army did a terrible job preparing leaders for the business aspects of medicine and needed to teach doctors about contracting and pay systems. Another believed that the Army was not adequately teaching soft skills (that this training needed to occur earlier than in the Army War College) and that better courses were needed to help clinical leaders understand "functional areas," such as how to "deal with congressmen" and how to conduct briefings.

As for methods, several respondents suggested tapping former leaders to provide the training, because they bring relevance and credibility. For example, as noted earlier, one leader described the executive skills training program as weak because "they don't have the relevant experience to talk to you about what you need to do." Another respondent believed that former commanders should be brought in to teach courses and that they needed to better utilize the capabilities of individuals who have had a lot of experience.

Respondents expressed mixed views about the value of online education. As noted earlier, several believed that attending the Army War College online removed the valuable experience of interacting and networking with other officers. However, others noted some benefits to online courses. One leader believed that online courses helped with self-education because some people feel freer to speak up and share their opinions in this format. Another respondent thought that more distance education options were needed for the Captain's Career Course because, without this option, not enough physicians had the opportunity to take the course.

Finally, two leaders believed that more frequent education was needed. One stated that more frequent exposure to the executive skills courses would benefit leaders. Another noted from personal experience that, given the rapid change occurring in the AMEDD, there were benefits to taking the course every few years, arguing that more "refresher courses" were needed.

Mentoring. Respondents agreed that mentoring was effective, but this opinion extended primarily to informal mentoring arrangements.

There was widespread agreement that mentoring was important for leader development (and most shared stories about how they were personally mentored at one point in their careers), but there were mixed views on how well the Army and AMEDD provided or fostered mentoring.

Many respondents identified mentoring as personally valuable for their own development and something to which they were personally committed. As one leader explained, "Whether it's been through just luck or maybe we're getting it, I've always had people that were mentors—but I've always sought the mentor." Another claimed to set aside one month each year to focus on mentoring in the organization and urged junior officers to "find a mentor and try to develop a relationship."

There was less agreement, however, on the extent to which the Army and AMEDD adequately provided this mentoring. Some felt that the Army was doing a good job in this area, noting that fewer leaders complained about a lack of mentoring and that more leaders had recognized mentoring as a key responsibility. A few noted that the OER system itself was supposed to be accompanied by mentoring, wherein the rater discusses the evaluee's career midterm, what is going well, and what he or she needs to work on. In fact, one leader mentioned sitting down monthly with those who were being evaluated to provide feedback and mentoring.

Others were far more critical. According to one leader, "We almost need a forced mentorship program; we are not mentoring our officers." That respondent noted, however, that part of the challenge in putting together mentoring programs was that few physicians had the command experience to serve as mentors to senior leaders. Another lamented that little face-to-face mentoring occurs and that there is an overreliance on emails. That respondent longed for the days when the branch chief would come to the clinics, sit down with officers, and "look them in the face and make them feel that they're important and that they are the most important person in their life."

One leader offered a different opinion about mentoring: "[I am] not a real fan of that mentoring push that is out there, because . . . a lot of people turn that into getting on someone's coattails and riding them." Instead, energy should be invested into ensuring that there are candid discussions about officers' performance and how they can improve.

Most respondents agreed that most mentoring occurred informally and that it was more effective this way. (A few dissented and wanted a mandated program.)

Many leaders reported that there was no formal mentoring system for medical leaders but that, in general, mentoring occurred voluntarily and informally. For example, several said that they self-selected mentors and role models. One leader explained, "I just chose my own mentors . . . because I wanted to be more like them and I saw them do things that I valued." This leader became a mentor in a similarly informal way and reported being sought out by others, adding, "I've never tried to force a mentoring relationship." Some respondents noted that they often serve as mentors but never explicitly label the relationships in this way. For example, one leader noted,

> I've mentored one specific officer from afar for the last several years, and though we've never formally discussed it, I know that we both feel that that's our relationship. She will call or email me out of the blue and run something by me, and we'll have a good little conversation about it, and that'll be the end of it for a few months. But I have identified her as a great junior officer and want to make sure that she is challenged and motivated in the right way because she's got so much potential.

Another respondent concurred: "*Mentor* is a term that is best ascribed and not assumed, so if it's ascribed to you by others, it's probably accurate. If you hear someone talking about how he is a mentor to others, that would make me suspicious."

While one person wanted the Army to mandate a mentoring program, most felt strongly that only informal mentoring could be effective. According to one leader, mentoring relationships develop through conversations and build organically: "The formality, I think, takes away from the whole process." Similarly, another was adamant that one cannot mandate mentoring and that such arrangements work only when they develop naturally over time.

Career Counseling. Respondents' views on career counseling included opinions about the need to self-select and the value of receiving such counseling early in one's career.

Some respondents cited the value of having received career counseling in their own careers, although they often noted that it was something they sought out on their own (self-selected rather than systematic development).

One leader recalled being a captain and sitting down with a supervisor to develop a career map that the respondent returned to many times over the years. This same leader acknowledged seeking out counseling and career advice from the various leaders for whom they had worked over the years. Another leader similarly recalled sitting down as a lieutenant with a mentor and preparing a 20-year plan that was broken down into five-year increments.

Although one leader reported that the branch chief and career managers regularly conducted one-on-one counseling, another said that this personal counseling occurred more in the past than it does now.

Some leaders identified a need for more career counseling early on in one's career.

One respondent acknowledged having "no idea these positions exist[ed]" early on and that it would be valuable to communicate and prepare officers early to think about their future. Similarly, another leader believed that officers needed assistance early in their careers to assess where they want to be in the future and whether they want to be commanders.

Feedback. Respondents valued anonymous 360-degree feedback, finding it helpful and honest.

A few mentioned the 360-degree evaluation process and feedback as a way of fostering leader development.

One leader explained that, as part of one ILE leader development cell, officers were encouraged to seek input from those for whom they had recently worked or for whom they had worked a long time ago. The respondent believed that, over time, these anonymous assessments helped reinforce individuals' perceptions of themselves and identify their strengths and weaknesses. Another leader mentioned the optional 360-degree online process offered through Army War College. This particular leader participated in the process and received a 110-page document with input from superiors, subordinates, and peers, characterizing it as "a real, pure look" that was not inflated. The leader described it as "one of the most useful documents I've had in leadership, because it included subordinates and peers and it was very helpful feedback. . . . I learned a lot about myself." The course instructor also spent about two hours reviewing the document with the respondent, which was also valuable.

Self-Development. Respondents reported a variety of opportunities for self-development, including online programs and reading lists.

A few respondents recognized the importance of self-initiated development for developing as a leader.

One respondent explained, "A fair part of that is independent education. All of the services are very much into reading programs, and self-teaching, and learning, and studying." Similarly, another leader described various "self-help" options for development, such as online courses and reading programs (e.g., Army Surgeon General and corps commander reading programs, division commander and brigade commander recommended readings), stating that they provide good foundations and research on various topics (e.g., strategic thinking): "Everything else is really self-development and self-tracked. So, it depends really on how motivated you are to develop your craft. No one's going to look over you and say, 'Did you read that?'"

How to Incentivize

Several respondents noted that various "development opportunities" greatly affected promotion and that the incentive of looking good when coming before boards and being considered for selection drives officers to seek out educational opportunities and new positions.

For example, one leader wanted to be a commander and needed certain skills. The leader also knew that attending a distance learning program through the Army War College and obtaining a master's degree would open up doors, noting that it was "practically a prerequisite . . . a discriminator when you go through those boards. . . . I recognize that the skills I learned would be necessary to do that job, but I also recognize that it's a discriminator for the board, so that's why I signed up."

Outcome

Several respondents held very positive views about the skills and abilities of current medical leaders.

Several respondents noted that AMEDD leaders had strong leadership skills, such as knowing how to be team players and being caring and inspiring. One leader believed that Army officers did well with "situational leadership styles" and knew how to match their leadership style to their environment. Finally, one leader believed that officers serving in joint staff assignments developed very strong skills and knew how to work well with other services.

Some respondents (five) noted weaknesses among clinical leaders.

Three non-MC leaders noted that physician leaders often struggled with leadership because they did not have as much training or grounding in certain skills due to their long investment in becoming clinically competent. One leader (MSC) explained, "At the very senior levels and at the general officer level, they're mostly physicians and they haven't had the experience set that many people at the lieutenant colonel, colonel levels have." The same respondent commented on their lack of experience:

> There are people in there selected for command that have not commanded anything. And here they are being now selected at the colonel level, and not only are they not commanding anything, . . . they have been department and service chiefs of 20, 30, 40, 50 people, which is commendable and important when you're a department chief or service chief of surgery, or a chief nurse of a hospital. But now, all of a sudden, instead of 50, 60, 100 people, I command today 2,800 people. It's a huge jump.

Similarly, another (MSC) leader commented,

> So we in the AMEDD, I think, have to do a better job of developing all officers to be commanders, if that's what they want to do. You can take a surgeon and put him in as a commander and they won't have the same skill sets. They're focused on patient care, where you have to be more open to your entire organization. . . . How do you train for briefings and [quarterly training brief] and MILCON development of your military construction projects? The whole gamut. . . . We have a pre-command course in the AMEDD, but it doesn't get to how do you deal with your sergeant major. What's the role of a sergeant major? Teaching them to be partners because out here, you've got to deal with the congressmen. [Physicians are] doing other things throughout their career, and then all of a sudden they come out on the command list. So I think we have to do a better job. The Medical Service Corps officers, no problems. There are a few docs who are exceptions because they go out and they become division surgeons. But those who stay within the AMEDD

and become department chiefs and that's all they've done, and now they're a commander—I just think we need to set them up for success.

A member of the NC also pointed to weaknesses among MC leaders:

It is a difficult task, because their focus—and I want this to be their focus—is their clinical practice. It is a difficult challenge out here in the field to give these young captain physicians the same type of experience. Actually, it is impossible to get them grounded in their basic leadership skills, because that is not their primary responsibility. As they then grow up, 20 years later, perhaps they will have acquired it along the way, but I just firmly believe that the due-course officer (Nurse Corps, Medical Service Corps) who has come in . . . and grown up in the Army over a career of two-and-a-half decades has that leadership base, and we are just so much better equipped because of it.

Finally, two other leaders—one a member of the MSC and the other a member of the MC—pointed to specific deficiencies in the area of business skills and knowledge. The MC leader, for example, believed that senior medical officers were not well prepared in "the business aspects of medicine" and needed to acquire skills in such areas as contracting, pay systems, and how to manage civilians. According to the MSC leader, clinical leaders needed to better understand "the business processes that go on in our systems."

Advice for Improving Leader Development

Many respondents argued that the Army and the AMEDD needed to identify potential leaders and provide development opportunities earlier in an officer's career.

As one leader stated, "We have to identify candidates early. It behooves us to identify them early, make them understand early we think they have potential, so they don't get out." Another respondent believed that junior officers needed strong mentorship early in their careers and that feedback should be offered and counseling should occur regularly, before officers are evaluated. Yet another argued for investing in educational opportunities earlier in an officer's career:

We need to send [them] for long-term schooling . . . earlier in their career. Brand-new majors or senior captains need to go. Don't be sending the senior majors or lieutenant colonels to these programs, because I think it's a waste of money. . . . Because they go to the program, they come back, they pay us back their two years and they get out of the Army. What you want to do is you want to send them in the middle when they're young, they're eager. . . . You get a longer return on your investment, and they use those skills in your organization.

Some respondents thought that training for COs should begin when an officer is a captain or major. As noted, some argued that clinical leaders should receive training during their residency program.

A few respondents offered suggestions for improving the selection process, such as improving OERs and board selection.

As noted earlier, several respondents suggested integrating an element of 360-degree evaluations into the official OER process by allowing for peer and subordinate input. Others simply argued for further training and time invested in writing evaluations to make these documents more meaningful. At least one wanted attention paid to the composition of the boards to ensure that they were not biased.

Two respondents implied that physicians needed more opportunities for leader development.

As one MC leader explained,

> From a Medical Corps perspective, I think what needs to be done is they need to give doctors the opportunity to participate. From the early part of my career, you never really had the opportunity to pull your nose off the patient care grindstone and indulge an interest in medical or health care management. You're not really afforded the same opportunity to do that as a care provider. That's not quite the same for the Nursing or Medical Services Corps. Their ability to move out of clinical duties and into some educational program or course is much more liberal. So, from a Medical Corps perspective, I think we need to focus a little more on after the doctor has done his residency and first three to four years of payback time and solidified his clinical skill sets, affording him the time to attend a four- or six-year-long course, like an [master of health administration] or whatever. I think that would do a lot to foster Medical Corps leaders.

Similarly, another MC officer argued that doctors should not be excluded from opportunities for leadership and leadership development.

Several leaders suggested ways to enhance leader development via job assignments and experiences.

One leader argued for the creation of a "leader intern" position to allow people to "try it on for size" before taking time out of their clinical lives to get an advanced degree. This leader also believed that it was important to recognize people for taking on such a position and making it a "little star on your [officer record brief]." Similarly, another leader believed that it was important to give potential leaders opportunities to "sit in a position" and have exposure to the responsibilities so that they are not experiencing the job for the first time when they are in charge. Several respondents also argued for earlier exposure and opportunities to lead, such as being put in charge of a committee or commission. Finally, one leader believed that SP officers deserved opportunities to be deputy commanders instead of going directly from department head to commanding officer positions. That respondent argued for opening up administrative lanes for SP officers.

Many respondents offered advice on how to improve education and training for leaders.

As noted earlier, several believed that clinical leaders needed more instruction on "the business aspects of medicine," such as budgets, contracts, and pay systems, and that, in the case of physicians, some of this instruction could occur during the residency program. One respondent also felt that clinicians needed more coursework on how to be a commander, such as how to work with Congress and give briefings. Others urged for increased opportunities for JPME and possible opportunities to integrate joint medical training, awareness, and cross-service training into existing courses. A few also suggested creating more fellowships and internships, while one leader wanted a distance learning option for the Captain's Career Course (to enable more doctors to participate). Several respondents argued for drawing on the expertise of former leaders to instruct leadership courses. Still others had suggestions about specific content, such as exposure to research on skills that define successful leaders, training on how to move back and forth between different types of jobs, and coursework on combatant command issues. (See the section on education and training under "How to Develop," earlier in this appendix.)

Findings from Interviews with Navy Health Professions Officers

The information in Appendixes C through E provided the input for the cross-case analysis reported in Chapter Four. This appendix presents the findings drawn from our interviews with Navy officers. This analysis draws mainly on 2008 interviews with respondents who were primarily MTF commanders. We also used material from the 2007 interviews, although they used a somewhat different protocol; not all were transcribed, and many were less comprehensive. We refer to all respondents in a gender-neutral way to ensure anonymity, but our sample included men and women as well as representatives from the different corps. As a reminder, at the beginning of the interviews, respondents were informed that when we asked about leader competencies and development, we meant executive-level health professions officers, such as the commander of an MTF, chief medical officer, CNO, and others at that level.

Context, Organizational Environment, and Organizational Leader Expectations

Context and Organizational Environment

Some interviewees (three) identified productivity expectations and pressures as important contextual factors that shape what is expected of leaders, who is selected, and how they are evaluated.

These respondents noted that, unlike in years past when medical officers were judged on how well they supported the forces and their families, there had been a movement in the past decade to evaluate medical leaders more on "the bottom line" and their contributions to productivity. As one commander explained,

> The only thing that's really changed in running a hospital in the military, I think, in the last ten years has been . . . you have to understand the business of medicine now. It's crucial, because we were never judged before on our ability to bring a product in, product per dollar. That was never in the mix. You were only judged by [what you] did [to] support the operational fighting forces. Did you take safe care

of the families that were entrusted to you? . . . And, if so, you're doing a great job. . . . They didn't care how many patients you saw, how many patients you didn't see, as long as the care was safe, and it was satisfying—and that the wartime fighters had no complaints. . . . But what's changed in the last ten years is that you can't survive now in running a medium- to big-sized military treatment facility unless you understand the business of medicine.

Several individuals described some of the unintended consequences of this shift. One believed that nurses were being moved into leadership positions so that doctors could continue seeing more patients to meet productivity demands. This individual believed that, as a result, doctors were not being properly developed for leadership roles. Similarly, another felt that the Navy was "reticent to remove them [doctors] from the clinical role simply because those are the guys who are generating the bucks." Thus, doctors may have to wait longer to get leadership positions. Others simply mentioned that these pressures had placed a premium on leaders gaining business-related skills and knowledge.

Three respondents identified a significant, more recent challenge to leading an MTF that related to the changing makeup of the staff, which now includes not only military personnel but also civilian and contract workers.[1]

According to these respondents, this diversity creates an environment in which individuals are working with different rules, goals, procedures, and expectations. One commander described their MTF as a "fragmented organization":

> You're dealing with three different systems. Often, you have military, civilian, and contractors, all of whom have different rules, have different goals, have different personnel structures and plans. And so, yes, these become much more fragmented than they used to be. And I think that's clearly an issue. . . . There's this larger turnover [with contractors]. You have little control.

This same respondent went on to explain how this fragmentation affected an MTF leader on a daily basis:

> It can come down to nothing more than before a holiday, I can tell the military personnel that they can leave early that day, if their work's done. [Similarly for] civilians. . . . [With a] contractor, I have to say, "I'm sorry. If you want to leave early, you'll have to do it without pay." I mean, something as simple as that, which doesn't seem like a lot. . . . Or, if people have done a good job, you can maybe let them out early. And [the contractors are] like, "Well, why are they getting the

---

[1] In some of the MTFs in our sample, civilians represented 25–50 percent of all staff and some top-level executive leaders (for example, chief information officer). Our interview sample consisted only of officers, however.

reward, and we're not?" Well, it's a different system. When it comes to planning training, if my military need training, it's very easy. I can set up a time. I can give them a place to be, and they're there. My civilians, if I work it into their [position descriptions], and I give them enough notice, I can change their work environment or have them come to training. Contractors: Is it written in their contract? . . . And who's going to pay for the training? Everything gets compounded. So it's not like you can just come up with an easy solution. When you think something should be easy, it often isn't. And that's a challenge.

Other respondents complained that Navy leadership development did not take into account the diversity of staff at the MTFs and the challenges this poses to leaders.

One respondent noted that, because of deployments, there is an incentive to staff certain positions with civilians to provide stability and "corporate continuity in product lines." According to this leader, "We'd rather deliberately set out to anchor some positions with civilians," particularly those that do not do well with "churn." However, several others noted potentially negative consequences of the new staffing arrangements that have occurred. In one MTF, deployments had left a very limited number of civil service employees to supervise contract workers. The large numbers of civilian workers in another MTF also had an adverse effect on the remaining military workers. For example, civilians are not allowed to perform many military-specific, collateral duties, such as serving on committees and watch. By converting more and more to civilian positions, this commander found that "there's really no one around to run those programs" and that the military workers are "working even harder."

Some respondents pointed to the new demands being made on leaders because of the need to work in joint environments, particularly interservice environments.

These demands call for new skills in working collaboratively with services that have different structures, different training, and different expectations. We discuss this further in the section on organizational leader expectations.

Some respondents (four) believed that retention problems and staff churn due to deployments were major obstacles to developing strong leaders.

Several leaders reported that deployments and conversions left MTFs understaffed and placed demands on clinicians that prevented them from seeking out other responsibilities and development opportunities. Others noted that the inability to retain staff due to the lure of industry and concerns about "quality of life" (frequent moves, deployments) affected the supply or pool of future leaders. For example, one reported,

I think one of the big challenges is retention. I think if you look at the distribution in terms of experience of the medical—I'll just talk to the Medical Corps, doctors—is that you have a whole bunch of junior people and people that just finished their residency. And you have a large bunch of senior people that are staying the 20, 30 years. But then, there's a big gap in the ten- to 16, eight- through 17-year period, when a lot of your lieutenant commanders and commanders are bailing. So I think that needs to be addressed. . . . They're the future leaders. And again, some people that do decide to stay in and make it a career, some of them don't have that potential to be a leader.

This same respondent lamented that there was only one doctor at their command that "showed potential" for becoming a leader.

Other leaders conveyed the flipside of this challenge: that retaining people and ensuring that individuals gain sustained experience contributes to leadership skills. For example, speaking from personal experience, one leader attributed his mentoring skills and the ability to develop others to length of experience as a leader:

You have to remember I'm on my second command tour. I've had two tours at headquarters. If you talk to other flag officers, you'll probably get this level of organized thinking. If you talk to people who are on their first CO tour, sometimes they're trying to figure it out. . . . It's something that I bring up with my subordinate COs. We talk about leader development, we talk about personal learning schedules, we talk about what you read and how you scan the environment and how you prevent inevitable or predictable surprises. These are the topics that I might be covering in one of my every-other-week meetings.

As a result, these leaders believed that it was essential for the Navy to stay competitive and attract and retain "good people."

Seven respondents noted the limited leadership and advancement opportunities in certain corps. These limitations were tied in some instances to the structural career paths in these corps.

Four respondents mentioned that NC members often did not get executive-level leadership opportunities until later in their careers, and, as a result, one noted, postcommand career options were very limited. As one respondent noted, the lack of postcommand opportunities meant that becoming a flag officer was "out of reach." Another member of the NC mentioned that because a limited number of officers can be promoted each year, regardless of performance, the corps is left with a pool of qualified personnel with nowhere to go.

There were mixed views on the leadership opportunities for MSC members. One respondent stated that these members had fewer leadership opportunities than officers in the other corps.

A few respondents believed that MC members and providers generally had more opportunities for leadership and command positions. However, several believed that because of the length of time required for clinical training and the demand to keep them in clinical positions (e.g., to meet productivity demands), it often took longer and was more difficult for these providers to gain the requisite skills and advance to leadership positions. Two respondents reported that the time frame of a doctor's career inhibited his or her opportunities to develop leadership and administrative skills. One noted that because of the length of time required to become a doctor, these individuals had little time to develop before they had to retire. Finally, one respondent identified a "glass ceiling" for certain positions (e.g., positions that do not oversee large numbers of people), such as "techies."

According to two respondents, a "rank-conscious" culture posed potential challenges to identifying and grooming talent in the Navy.

As one leader explained,

> We do tend at times to be very rank-conscious and reticent to step outside of that structure and say, "Okay, I'm going to name this O-3 to be the division head over these O-4s because I think [he or she is] a better performer and I think [he or she] can do the job more efficiently than the O-4s." I would say that rank is there for a reason, but it shouldn't be held up as the [be-all and] end-all of everything.

Similarly, another commander believed that the most significant challenge faced by the Navy in identifying and supporting high-potential officers was "being stuck in the way they've always done it." That respondent went on to explain that the military follows a "rank paradigm for leading."

Leader Expectations

As was true of the other two services, although most Navy respondents were asked how the Navy defines an ideal leader, many responded by providing their opinions about what they felt were important characteristics or criteria for leaders.

Many respondents (seven) emphasized experience as critical for identifying and defining a leader.

In answering the question of how the Navy defines an ideal leader, many respondents cited certain positions or a career progression that often emphasized more than a particular set of traits, skills, or knowledge. For example, one commander responded that an ideal leader was someone who had done well in different assignments, while another said it was someone who had demonstrated success in leadership at various levels. In fact, many stressed the importance of accumulating a breadth of experience. Some felt that this meant having exposure to a wide range of billets. Others felt that it meant having operational and deployment experience. As one commander explained, leaders needed "experience in doing something similar at a smaller command. . . .

Something that would have exposed them to all the intricacies of managing a medical center."

Most respondents, representing the spectrum of corps, believed that leaders should possess and maintain clinical skills—particularly for the credibility such skills bring.

Many noted that keeping up one's clinical skills is important for "the acceptance of all the people that you're leading," as one commander put it. Another said that clinical competency was "taken as a given." At least one respondent believed that a leader's greatest credibility came from being an MC provider. This respondent noted that older generations, in particular, wanted to be led by a practicing provider, not a nurse or MSC member: "It's very tough for them to suddenly have a nurse come in when they've been used to doctors running things." Others believed that maintaining at least a limited clinical practice helps a leader understand what occurs throughout the MTF. One respondent (MC) noted,

> It also keeps you in touch with the organization. If you're never seeing patients, you've kind of lost track of what you're there for in some ways or lost the reality of the day to day. So for me, at least, it's useful to be able to continue to see patients.

Similarly, another leader (MC), explained, "It's critical that you maintain your credentials . . . also [so] that you have some idea of what's going on."

A few respondents were pragmatic about the importance of maintaining clinical skills, acknowledging that "you don't know when you'll need them" (e.g., post-command). At least one respondent cautioned, however, that clinical skills are not sufficient and do not always translate to leadership skills. According to this leader (MC),

> I think there are certain things about your clinical ability that need to be looked at. . . . It's one thing if I am the fastest surgeon and I can do hernias or take out somebody's gallbladder really quick. But it's another thing if I'm that kind of surgeon and I just treat everybody in the OR [operating room] horribly. And so I think that there are certain things that do translate. . . . Like, clinically speaking, if I direct my clinical effort to improving patients, they see an elevating standard care for patients and I do things beyond the OR to make those kind of things happen instead of just spending my time in the OR, then, yes, I think that is something that translates to someone who has leadership potential. But if you just look at somebody strictly for their technical ability and you don't see how they use their technical ability to help expand the entire clinical environment, then maybe they don't have leadership skills.

Finally, several respondents noted the challenge of maintaining clinical skills while also fulfilling their many other leadership duties.

Several respondents (five) cited the importance of leaders having business and management skills, while a few clarified that leading is not the same as managing.

In several interviews, leaders mentioned that executive-level health professions officers needed a strong understanding of the "business of medicine," including financial and human capital management. One leader described these areas as "the didactics of leadership" and noted that they were measured well by Navy fitness reports and taken into account during the process of selection. Several were quick to note that managing is not the same as leading. As one respondent explained,

> We expect our midgrade officers to be good managers. They need to be able to manage their immediate resources and their staff. As you get to be a leader, it's a matter of being able to not only manage your day to day, but to be able to look over your entire organization, to be able to utilize your resources appropriately, to be able to determine what it is that you need to do to meet the mission, and to also . . . be able to look strategically downstream and say not only how are you meeting the mission today, but how are you going to be meeting the mission in five years?

Similarly, another leader noted,

> I guess you can teach anyone to be a manager, and we distinguish between the managers and the leaders. You have to be a good manager if you're going to be in a supervisory position, or we move you out of that position. As far as being a leader, all my supervisors and all my managers are not leaders.

According to several respondents (six), leaders need "enterprise" knowledge, skills, and abilities, such as strategic thinking and being awareness of the larger environment. Some also included political skills in their descriptions.

As noted earlier, several Navy respondents identified skills that went beyond traditional organizational management to include facets of what we considered "enterprise" knowledge, skills, and abilities, or what respondents described as "systems-level thinking," understanding the whole organization, being "strategic," and knowing how to "set a vision." One respondent described such leaders as "mature decisionmakers with systems-level thinking ability" who can "think ahead, . . . find the next surprise before it hits you in the face, . . . [and] understand risk and operational or organizational risk management." Several others added to this an expectation of being politically savvy. For example, one respondent noted that leaders needed to be "politically aware of what is the current environment and the administration in the military to be able to understand the environment that you're operating in," adding,

> And so what, generally, . . . they're looking for is someone who's able to say, "Okay, these are the strategic goals of the Navy overall and Navy medicine." And this is

the path that they perceive that they want us to go down. And so it's being able to take all of that input and then be able to manage whatever's under your control as a leader to get it there.

Similarly, another leader explained,

I think the admiral would look for political astuteness, someone who has an understanding of the importance of what we do, appreciates . . . the significance of being in [Washington, D.C.] and the fact that, as you've found at Walter Reed, everything you do is a front-page news story.

Several (six) respondents believed that the softer aspects of leadership were also very important, such as possessing strong interpersonal skills and knowing how to develop others.

In several interviews, respondents noted that a set of less didactic or technical skills—described as "soft" or "intangible"—were very important for leadership. Some highlighted the value of being able to work on a team and build strong teams, mentor and develop subordinates, and create consensus. As one explained, a leader needs to develop troops and "empower them to be able to do what they need to do." Interestingly, there was some disagreement about the extent to which the Navy valued and formally recognized the importance of these aspects of leadership. One individual felt strongly that they were frequently overlooked:

We don't, oftentimes, evaluate an individual on the other, intangible qualities of leadership. You know, their interpersonal skills, their own self-awareness, their ability to create consensus or to be able to understand what works when you're trying to create change—what that represents for the different people you're trying to lead. We don't really have a way of assessing that, measuring that, and nor do we necessarily recognize that in people.

In contrast, several respondents believed that a leader's ability to mentor and develop others was a very important and formally evaluated aspect of leadership. One leader explained,

Mentorship is a big deal to us. We use it usually as one of our criteria when evaluating people and their performance . . . how well they're mentoring their junior people, how well they're developing them. How well are their people under them being promoted? How well are their people under them getting jobs of greater responsibility?

Four respondents referred to educational background and knowledge as important criteria for leaders.

While most emphasized the importance of advanced degrees or completion of particular courses, a few also noted that it was important for leaders to demonstrate academic success or knowledge.

Other criteria or aspects of leadership identified as important included the following:

- *Character and commitment:* One respondent believed that leaders needed to be fair, demonstrate integrity, and offer to "give 100 percent"; another believed that leaders at this level needed to be highly committed to what they do.
- *Flexibility:* One respondent said that leaders needed to be willing to move around.
- *Diversity:* One respondent felt strongly that leaders needed to embrace diversity:

Do they have a foundation and an understanding of equal opportunity and of diversity? Do they lead by example in those areas? Do they embrace diversity? Do they understand not only the moral implications of being and embracing diversity, but do they understand the strategic implications to an organization of embracing diversity?

- *Navy competency:* Respondents cited the need to understand the Navy command structure and policies.
- *Understanding of information systems:* Respondents noted that it was important to be familiar with information systems and how to use them to make more informed decisions.

Most respondents attested to the value of joint experience and education but were reluctant to make them mandatory.

In most interviews, we asked respondents their opinions about the extent to which executive leaders needed joint experience and education and whether they believed that these requirements should be made mandatory. Several noted that, because the military has been heading toward joint operations, it is important for officers to gain exposure to and learn about the language, systems, tools, and other features of all the services. In fact, many respondents gave examples of situations in which joint knowledge and skills would be particularly valuable. For example, one leader reported,

We go to war, and we pull some guy out of a med center, out of a hospital, never been in the Marine Corps, and say, "Run the medical for this echelon 3 situation right now in Iraq," or someplace, and that's what happens. . . . They haven't the faintest idea of how the Marine Corps works, what it does, how it thinks. . . . You get less than the capability you need. . . . Joint gives you that. So when I was in [country to which respondent was deployed], and I had to worry about tantamount [concerns], and I had to worry about Air Force MedEvac and all, I had no experience. I'd been totally Navy and Marine Corps, but Marine Corps happens to have air, happens to do joint stuff. I had a little knowledge that I could use. . . . I was able to be better than what you might expect, . . . but it would help if you had some better credentials and qualifications and knew how that service and everything works. . . . Medicine is trying to become more joint, as it is to get more joint programs. . . . And the services, . . . they just do it their way, even though you've made this agreement. . . . [The Army] took care of this patient, they had him on anesthesia, they had tubes and all. [He] came to the Air Force to MedEvac, and guess what, the tubes and all didn't match what . . . the Air Force had, so now you have to make those changes. So those are the kind of things we're trying to work through.

In contrast, one leader stood out for having a slightly different perspective on the necessity of joint experience and training: Not all medical officers needed this preparation. According to this respondent, medical officers needed to be clinically prepared and trained, and this was the most effective use of training dollars.

Many respondents were aware of a set of formal leadership competencies endorsed by the military, but most did not remember the acronym (JMESP) and tended to think of them as perfunctory "boxes you check off" in order to get promoted.

Few respondents mentioned these competences without solicitation. When probed about particular competencies that the Navy expects from leaders (often a follow-up to another question about how the Navy defines an ideal leader), many respondents referred to the list of 40 (now 39) competencies but often did not remember the source or acronym. Most of these respondents did not view these competencies as particularly meaningful or consequential. As one leader explained,

Would somebody not be selected for a leadership position that hadn't made sure they ticked all the boxes? I don't think that's the case, but on the other hand, I think most of us, when we were coming up through the ranks, felt that it was important that we tried to tick as many of those boxes as we could.

Most respondents also seemed to characterize these competencies as something you "get" or "obtain," not demonstrate. One leader noted that there was no standardized method for determining whether people gained these competencies. Another explained that officers submit to the system that they have "achieved" the competencies through a variety of experiences, but this reporting did not guarantee or demonstrate that officers have mastered the competencies.

Approach to Leader Development

Although our interview protocols and questions emphasized leader development—how and when individuals are identified for leader development opportunities—respondents often answered by describing who was selected as a leader and when. This likely had to do with how they and the services define leadership development: Much depends on experience (i.e., giving someone the opportunity to lead and gain on-the-job experience to develop them as a leader). As a result, the following themes blend both areas: identifying leaders and identifying individuals for leader development.

Like the other services, the Navy does have a purposeful system for identifying high-potential officers, although *some respondents were critical of the "lock-step" approach.* One believed that the Navy's "lock-step" requirement that an individual needed to be a director, then an XO, then a CO overlooked other opportunities for individuals to develop skills, demonstrate their potential, and be selected.

> I would argue that leadership and leadership skills are being manifested in a lot of different areas of the enterprise, and if we don't sensitize ourselves and school ourselves to look across the spectrum, then all we're going to be doing is looking at the people who go through [the] department head/director/XO/CO [route]. And we lose out on that opportunity to get people out there who are incredibly courageous, very creative, and extremely self-aware and very self-confident, to be able to go out to where the resistance is the greatest and find out, okay, what is it that is creating this for you?

> When we get so locked into [the] department head/director/XO/CO [route] . . . we oftentimes don't see these other opportunities that are out there that help not only develop those skills but also help the individual demonstrate their ability. And so, part of what I feel that I need to do is encourage some of my people. . . . As an example, somebody came the other day and they said, "Well, you know, all the director's jobs are taken. I want to be able to —." . . . And I said, "Well, you know, you don't need to look at the director's job; here are all these other things that can get done." But it was hard for him to appreciate that these opportunities showcased his talent or [gave] him what he thought he needed on the fitness report so he could be promoted or be considered for the job.

Some leaders (four) characterized the Navy's approach to leader development as happenstance or lacking purposeful planning and design.

In several interviews, the notion of "luck" or "serendipity" entered into the description of how the Navy prepares and develops its leaders. For example, one leader stated that one can look at any class of officers and say, "Well, one or two of those were a star, happened to get a mentor, and they brought everybody else along." Another leader noted that there was "an element of luck" to the process of identifying, assigning, and developing leaders in terms of "what's available at the right time." Still another identified some improvement in this area, noting that the Navy had become more thoughtful about training and equipping leaders with what they needed. However, this leader admitted that the Navy was still not as clear or as proactive as it could have been about identifying individuals early and "heading them down a codified path for leadership":

> We do not identify our people early enough in their pipeline to get them groomed for training. If it happens, it happens, sort of—either by people serendipitously follow[ing] the right track or they happen to luck into somebody who kind of grabs them by the shoulders and says, "This is what I want you to start doing at this point in your life." . . . We do it a little better in the Medical Service Corps and in the Nurse Corps, but in the Medical Corps, there's just a lot more haphazard nature to it.

In fact, several respondents noted that the Army did this better by providing a much more "scripted" and "prescribed" path, delineating the education and training that was required for those taking on leadership positions.

One respondent, who stated that development occurred in a "haphazard" manner, noted the following: First, individuals who are not qualified to lead are often selected because other, more qualified candidates are deployed; second, too much learning is expected to occur on the job; and third, who receives development opportunities such as mentoring and coursework depends heavily on "serendipity."

In contrast, one respondent described a more purposeful process and had already identified a successor.

This commander explained,

> I'm a subordinate, so somebody's developed me. My director, my deputy commander here, it's his responsibility and his task order to make sure that I'm prepared to take the next stepping stone. And I think that's something we do in the military real well, is we always look at two things. I'm trying to work myself out of a job. I'm trying to prepare the person underneath me to take my job, and I know that they're ready when they're doing my job and I'm just sitting here doing nothing. Likewise, I'm trying to take the next higher job up. I'm looking at either becoming a director of all the clinics or a deputy commander or an XO somewhere, so they're developing me and doing the same things with that.

Some respondents characterized the Navy's overall approach to identifying individuals for leadership and leader development opportunities as overly subjective.

For example, one believed that the process relied too heavily on "who you know." Another felt that the criteria for selecting leaders varied and depended significantly on who sat on the selection board. That respondent explained that the same individual could be passed up several times by the board and then get selected when the makeup of the selection board changed.

Two respondents believed that the process of identifying leaders had not paid adequate attention to promoting diversity.

One leader observed that the military had not made an adequate commitment to ensuring diversity among its leaders, not only in terms of gender and race but also "diversity of mind" and viewpoints:

> I think that's the one challenge that people have in leadership is do you want to grow an organization that looks like you, or do you truly want a diverse, dynamic organization that can adapt and move into the future?

Similarly, another leader commented on the homogeneity of leadership and believed that, although some attention was being paid to diversity, not enough was being done to change patterns: "If we keep on bringing in the same people who are going through the same process, we're going to end up with the same output, the same product."

Many respondents (seven) reported that the time frame when individuals were offered leader development opportunities was often either too early or too late.

These comments raised a question: At what point does it makes sense to introduce leader development opportunities? At least one leader suggested that if they are offered too early in a career, the individual has no experience to which he or she can apply the new knowledge: "Back when they did send me to the formal school, there was a lot of it that was not that important to me at the time." However, others indicated that, if delayed too long, the information and learning may no longer be useful or simply repeat what is already known or learned from experience. In fact, six leaders indicated that formal development opportunities often came too late. Several respondents mentioned that they wished they had received some of their development opportunities earlier in their careers. For example, one leader was adamant that the Navy needed to be more proactive in providing opportunities to individuals before they are in leadership positions, rather than offering them "after the fact."

This leader went on to explain how various financial, legal, and management courses would have been valuable if taken prior to promotion to a leadership position because they could have provided a better framework to answer pertinent leadership questions: "What do I need to ask about? What are higher-level people looking at?" Similarly, another respondent was critical of the timing of JPME: "I think that the wrong time, again—and this is how 90 percent of us are learning about joint—is the first time we're thrown into a joint environment. That's the wrong time to really learn about the vocabulary in the Army or the vocabulary in the Air Force." Another was critical of an assumption that individuals can learn business skills on the job and believed that formal training was necessary before taking on a leadership position: "You can't afford to learn that for the first time when you take over one of these organizations."

Several other respondents acknowledged that, often, the "timing doesn't work out" because certain courses are oversubscribed, not enough slots are available, or individuals are forced to take on a new position quickly, and, as a result, individuals cannot get into the course until after they have taken on the new position for which the course is intended to prepare them.

Again, much of these discussions pertained to selecting leaders, not identifying leaders for development.

How to Select

Most respondents (eight) reported that fitness reports were the primary method of identifying individuals with leadership potential, but many viewed them as subjective and noted that informal processes of identifying leaders and potential leaders often trumped the formal ones.

Leaders generally described the fitness reports as one of the primary formal means of identifying individuals for leadership positions and nominating them for various leader development opportunities. However, most were quick to note the limitations of these reports. One respondent characterized this as the "say-do gap," in which the report "may be glowing, but in reality, the individual may not have a skill set that aligns with what I need." Another leader provided a detailed, hypothetical example illustrating the subjectivity involved in the process:

> It's going to be very individualistic. And that's the difficulty of the system, even when it comes to the fitness report, which is supposed to be an objective assessment. To give you an example, you have Lieutenant Smith. Lieutenant Smith works for . . . Commander Jones. And Jones doesn't happen to like extroverts. And Lieutenant Smith is actually an extrovert and very good with her patients, and actually gets a lot done. But Commander Jones doesn't perceive it as such, because they're an introvert, and [he] thinks they're wasting time talking to other individuals that work there or that they're too loud or too assertive. But in fact, they're not only getting their job done, they're getting more than their job done, and they're creating a network. And it's actually facilitating their job. But Commander Jones doesn't perceive that. So when Lieutenant Smith's fitness report is done, [she is] perhaps not given the higher score in leadership, or it's worded in such a way that it almost potentially [minimizes] that person. Conversely, you have the opposite. Commander Jones is, as you know, not even assertive, but kind of a

friendly, outgoing-type person, if they're not extroverted. And Lieutenant Smith is an introvert. And Lieutenant Smith gets a lot of work done but really doesn't like to engage [with] other people or is very detail-oriented, while Commander Jones is a big-picture person and thinks this person's nitpicking and quiet and hangs in their office and [Commander Jones] doesn't appreciate the fact that they've rewritten three regulations, and looked at the process and refined it, and done a lot of work. So that's never reflected in their fitness report. And neither one of those people is ever then sent forward, even though both may have equal potential to be leaders in different ways. And that's a fault in our system.

Nevertheless, many respondents seemed to acknowledge that, regardless of the limitations, the fitness reports were valuable: "The fitness report, as subjective as it is, it does provide some objective basis for the decisionmakers to decide, 'Yes, this person's doing what they need to be doing and this person's not.'" Others simply noted that they had learned to "read between the lines" and identify "cues" in the text to uncover a true assessment of individuals.

Finally, others believed that because of these limitations, many decisions relied more on informal sources, such as discussions among leaders, particularly for more senior positions. "As they move up into the more . . . senior executive roles," explained one respondent, "fitness reports, . . . in my personal opinion, play less of a role as does service reputation and word of mouth." Similarly, when asked whether there was a process by which high-potentials were identified for leadership, one leader said, "Not really. They'll tell you all kinds of them, [but] there's none really. It's kind of, 'You know what you are.'" Others concurred that reputation and informal conversations often served as the basis for identifying potential leaders.

Two individuals mentioned being interviewed for positions and indicated that this may be increasing throughout the Navy.

One commander explained,

The interesting thing that we started doing recently in the Navy is interviewing for these positions. There were 13 people that interviewed for the position that I'm in. . . . I'd never interviewed for anything in my life. . . . So, we actually had to interview and put together a CV, sit before a board, the whole bit. So it wasn't as simple as saying, "This is your next assignment." It's really a selection, again, a competitive selection and who is the best fit and who's going to make the most impact on this position. [Interviewer: "And what's the rationale for the shift to interviewing as opposed to assigning?"] I think just that. Not only is the competition a good thing for the Navy, it's another way for us, them, however you want to read that, to identify people who are going to be at the higher-performing level.

Another leader explained that any admiral who was serious about what he or she was doing would use personal interviews to fill positions and not rely entirely on detailers' advice.

How to Develop

Job Assignments and Experiences. Overall, respondents had mixed views of the Navy's approach to job assignments and leader development.

Some respondents (four) characterized the Navy's approach to leader development as development "by fire," in which individuals are thrown into leadership positions and expected to acquire the necessary skills on the job.

As one leader explained, "We do have certain courses we have to take, . . . but there's not a formal leadership development. You get it basically by doing the jobs." Similarly, when asked whether the Navy had programs to give technically skilled individuals (e.g., doctors) training before they assumed executive positions, another leader responded, "They're just thrown in there and the assumption is that you're going to try to acquire it." Another concurred that this was a particular challenge for the MC:

> [It] is the same problem that the country has, and that is that you're a great doc, you're the best in your field, you can do the best care in the world, you can run your department and all, [and] suddenly we anoint you, make you an XO, you go in [trial by fire] for two years, and since we've already anointed you, we just figure out how good you are, and how good you are determines which level of MTF you get. But then you're right at the MTF, and what do we ask of you? We ask you to be a comptroller, we ask you to be a magician with material management, facilities, base ops, a business manager, a mentor, a coach, disciplinarian; you're going to have captain's mask, so you're going to be legal, and a judge, and all that stuff. And you get that kind of by fire for two years as an XO, and then we anoint you, and you go do it. And since we have fantastic medical people that did it in residency, became the best surgeons and doctors in the world, guess what, you don't see all the drop-offs and problems that would create in normal things, because they're exceptional people. But you really don't get trained; you don't really get to go through those steps. Now, MSCs get a little of that.

Another leader was less critical of this approach and noted that, because leadership is so difficult to teach or train, development occurs most effectively when people are given opportunities to lead and then are provided with feedback and mentoring.

While some leaders were critical of the Navy's emphasis on on-the-job training, others saw it as a valuable, planned strategy to provide people with increasing responsibility and to broaden their experiences.

As noted earlier, many respondents commented on the emphasis the Navy places on on-the-job training for developing leaders. Whether they were critical or supportive, most described a system by which individuals were given opportunities to experience increasing levels of responsibility and scopes of work, both preparing them with the knowledge and skills to lead and providing exposure to what leadership positions entail. One commander noted that certain staff positions allowed people to gain more experience and exposure. For example, this individual took on a policy-level position at one point, which provided a "very good overview of the bigger enterprise and what executive medicine would be like." The commander noted that others took on detailer positions or positions in Health Affairs to determine whether they were interested in leadership. In fact, an admiral advised this individual to take the policy-level position before taking on an XO position. The rationale was that such decisions help a potential leader ensure that he or she likes a particular type of work before making a move and potentially putting strain on his or her family. Another leader used assignments as a purposeful way to develop people:

> I'm looking at my directors. . . . Are they ready to be a chief operating officer? If they're not, what's the developmental experience they still need? So, for example, two of my directors I just deployed because they didn't have senior operational experience.

Two respondents mentioned collateral duties as another means of developing leaders. These duties, such as serving on or chairing a committee, were viewed as a useful way to provide clinical staff with leadership experience and exposure to "the administrative side of things" while still allowing them to remain in their clinical positions.

Many leaders described a common career path to becoming an MTF commander or executive. There were mixed views about how well this approach identified and fully developed leaders with potential. Several were critical of its rigidity and limitations, while at least one thought that more prescription was needed to adequately prepare leaders.

Many respondents described a similar trajectory in terms of how individuals moved up the ladder, gaining increasing responsibility over time. For example, many noted that one becomes a department head, director, XO, and then perhaps a leader of a small MTF, then a commander of a larger MTF. As noted earlier, one respondent described this as a "lock-step career path" and felt that it was too rigid.

However, another leader believed that the Navy needed to do a better job of "codifying the process" of how individuals move into "bigger jobs." That respondent noted, for example, that the Navy often put people into CO jobs when their only experience was as an XO or CO of a very small facility or clinic. Thus, they "sink or swim very quickly. They get overwhelmed. And then some do well." The respondent believed that serving as a deputy commander or XO of a region or medical center should be a prerequisite for taking charge of such an organization:

> Unless you've had to cut your teeth on high senior jobs in those areas first, the learning curve can be pretty steep. And so I think what happens is that it doesn't mean you won't be successful. It just means you can't hit the ground running, and so you spent the first six months to a year just learning your way around the organization, and then you can make your changes.

Although several leaders valued joint assignments, most were uncomfortable making them mandatory.

As noted earlier, several respondents pointed to the value of joint assignments and people who were experienced in working across services and agencies. However, most of these respondents believed that, while essential, it did not make sense to make joint assignments (and education) mandatory for advancement because there were not enough spots or billets. One leader stated, "My gut feeling says . . . because there are so few jobs, that you would lose some quality people."

Education and Training. Respondents cited a variety of sources for education and training, but they pointed to several barriers to pursuing these opportunities.

Most respondents cited various Navy-sponsored courses and programs that they had taken or were required to take over the course of their careers, including some online courses. Several also mentioned conferences.

Most simply described the content of these opportunities. Two respondents noted that some of the content of this training and education tended to be tied to the larger needs of the Navy. For example, one noted a strong emphasis on human capital management in recent years. Another described the progression over the years from a focus on management to Total Quality Management and, now, Lean Six Sigma. That respondent explained it as "the black belt, and green belt, and blue belt, whatever it is. So sort of as you grow, you do whatever the interest is of your service."

A few respondents commented on the perceived value of these internal courses. For example, one leader realized a need for more background in finance and legal matters and sought out these courses while a director. Although the leader found them to be valuable, the impression was that they would have been useful earlier on. Similarly, another leader who sought out various "leadership courses" noted that they were "most helpful" in "validating some of the things that I thought might be more effective" and giving "a little better perspective on how I might expand on my current effort or where I was."

Several other respondents were critical of the lack of supply or access to some opportunities (e.g., demand for business education courses outstripped supply, no training for commanders, limited seats in interagency and capstone courses). A few wanted more training for civilians. One wanted more education and training on how to manage the different civilian, military, and contract systems and workers in MTFs. Another leader felt that courses could use more editing and that content spread across ten days could easily be covered in two days.

Several respondents were critical of joint education, particularly the amount of time it took to complete.

Several noted that it took too much time to complete the senior service and war college courses. One leader said that it was especially difficult for doctors to drop what they are doing and results in a loss of their bonus. Many were also concerned about the limited number of spots available in these programs. Several respondents believed that the military needed to come up with another option—for example, training tailored to military leaders that would familiarize them with how the other services work, or infusing some of this education into existing, standard courses.

Another felt strongly that all programs should be conducted online. Finally, one respondent stressed that those who were selected for war college did not always apply what they learned to their subsequent positions, because the Navy is not deliberate in how it assigns individuals after they attend these programs:

> We don't always utilize these people to the best advantage. . . . It's not a real codi-fied process. Sometimes, the seats come open. And the assignment officer gets a phone call from [the Industrial College of the Armed Forces] or the National War College or the Air Force Staff College or the Marine Staff College. And they say, "Hey, we've got some seats. And we'd like—we can't fill them. Would you guys like them?" And our guys go, "Yeah, yeah, that'd be great. What a great opportunity for a nurse or for a doc." And so they send something. They say, "Hey, Schmedly, we don't know what to do with you, you know? You were a department head in Guam. And you want to be in executive medicine. But we don't have any big jobs open for you now. So we want you to go back and see patients." And Schmedly says, "Ahh, I don't want to see patients. I kind of like this executive stuff." "But we got a seat at the war college. Want to go do that?" "Yeah, that sounds cool." So they go to the war college. They do that for a year. And then they come out of the war college all pumped up with all this information and doctrine and policy and engagement issues and understanding humanitarian assistance and all that. And they go to their detailer and they say, "Okay, where can you play me now? Should I go be in charge of a fleet medical department?" And [the] detailer says, "No, no. I have a burning need that's come up over the last year for a executive offi-cer in Corpus Christi, Texas." And they go, "You just spent a fortune educating me on what the Chinese are doing and North Koreans, and how we're going to build this, and how to build a task force to combat cholera and malaria." "Yeah, yeah, yeah, yeah, yeah. But I need you in Corpus Christi, Texas." . . . So we do that all

the time, all the time. So there's this mismatch. We don't preordain what's going to happen with these people.

Several respondents (five) identified the value of education and training opportunities provided by individuals and organizations outside of the military.

In many cases, these outside opportunities were sponsored by the Navy (e.g., master's programs). One leader believed that, at the senior executive level, most individuals sought courses outside the military because the military did not provide equivalent opportunities. This leader was particularly appreciative of courses taken from the ACHE. Another respondent was more critical of the military's approach to adult education and sought out external courses as a result of this perceived weakness:

> Proportionally, the military doesn't understand adult learning too well. We understand it for our lines, like pilots and submariners and all, but we're all adult learners, which [means] we don't want to learn something unless we're going to have real implementation of something that's going to be of benefit to us. . . . You're going to have to really talk about a whole program concept to present it, and then you start with, "What are the building blocks to get there?" You can't have this unless you have that. And why is that element of learning or capability critical to what you're doing? . . . Residency training in medicine does that, it's one of the best, it's always been that way, it's why people go crazy to get in.

Two respondents reported that lack of time was a barrier to participating in formal education and training.

As one leader explained, "At the senior level, many don't have the time" to enroll in educational offerings like a master's program. As a result, in the leader's opinion, these master's programs would never be a "major pathway" for development or a "major tool in my quiver." Another noted that the time commitment for attending war college was a problem.

One leader mentioned two other constraints to participating in training.

First, officers hesitate to attend the Joint Trauma Care Course because the perception is that completion leads to deployment in Iraq. Second, the leader noted that dentists are in short supply, so it is difficult to send them to leadership training.

Mentoring. As in the Army, mentoring in the Navy is characterized mainly by informal arrangements, according to our respondents.

Many interviewees (eight) mentioned informal mentoring they had received over the years and generally characterized mentoring in the Navy as informal in nature.

As one commander explained, "We formally talk about it. It informally happens. And again, typically how that happens is kind of individual initiative." Another described benefiting from informal mentors:

> I have at least two or three people that have . . . mentored me. And each time, they provide you some of that feedback and the guidance on what jobs to take or what collaterals to take or what areas you need to work on.

Two respondents felt strongly that mentoring was not successful when it occurred formally. "When it becomes formal," said one leader, "often, those who don't really want to be doing it—whether as a mentor or mentee—aren't fully participatory. And so the results aren't as productive as people would like." Another leader explained,

> A mentor relationship, it can't be an assigned thing. . . . Sometimes, you don't click and it doesn't work. It really has to be kind of a mutual, agreed-upon thing and . . . in my experience, that happens . . . as you're working in the area like where I am right now. I may look across several directorates or at several other people in jobs above me and say, "This person is someone who I feel comfortable working with," and I'll approach them, talk to them, or they may contact me and say, "Hey, I notice we've got similar interests. Your career path that you look like you're going down is similar to mine," and you establish a relationship in that way. But to dictate it and say, "This is going to be your mentor"—that sounds very military, but that's not really the way we do it.

One respondent, however, felt that formal mentoring was preferable to informal mentoring, arguing that formal mentoring ensured less sporadic interactions and provided for greater communication. Nevertheless, like the others interviewed, this individual believe that it was critical for the person being mentored to opt into the relationship.

Career Counseling. Career counseling was rarely discussed during interviews with our Navy respondents.

Although career counseling occurred regularly in a formal way, few respondents brought it up or discussed it as a formal leader development strategy.

Only one respondent mentioned midterm counseling with the Career Development Board, in which officers talk with more senior officers about career goals and steps necessary to reach them.

Feedback. The concept of 360-degree feedback was brought up less frequently than in our Army interviews, but one respondent reported that it was growing in popularity.

A few respondents mentioned the concept of 360-degree evaluations.

Interestingly, only one leader mentioned the Navy's 360-degree evaluation program but thought it had "taken off" in past couple of years. That respondent described the process of submitting names of several subordinates, colleagues, and superiors who were then contacted and given series of questionnaires. (The respondent did not comment on and was not probed on the perceived value of receiving this feedback.) One commander had participated in a 360-degree process as part of an ACHE course and noted the value of this feedback:

> [It] gave you feedback on your own leadership style, your management style, how others perceived you. So when you were able to sit and look at that, you had all of that ready for you when you came to the class. So, not only did you learn about all the different leadership styles and team building and ways to move an organization forward, but you then had some concrete feedback that you had in your hand that showed, really, a little bit more about yourself. . . . I'm not sure if the cost would make it worthwhile or not. But it was . . . [a way to] if nothing else . . . reaffirm or not your own belief. Frankly, sometimes people think they're one thing, and they're not.

The commander also noted, "It's always nice to know what your boss thinks of you, but what does your staff really think of you? What do your peers think of you?"

Self-Development. According to respondents, it was necessary for potential leaders to seek out development opportunities on their own.

Many respondents (seven) noted that many development opportunities, particularly at the top executive levels, were self-initiated: Individuals sought out classes and opportunities on their own, often in an effort to make themselves more "promotable."

When describing their own career paths, most leaders characterized their decision to pursue a particular development opportunity (e.g., obtaining a master's degree, attending a particular course) as self-initiated and not something that was recommended or required. Several leaders emphasized that individuals in the military had to take responsibility for seeking out development opportunities. "There are courses out there," said one leader. "But you have to go and actively ask for them." Another leader commented,

> If you feel like you're struggling, you're having difficulty in one particular area— let's say budgeting or personnel—depending on what level you're at, I think it's incumbent upon the person in that position to seek out help, and it's available out there. It will be recognized eventually that you've got shortfalls in that area, and if you don't do something about it before it comes to the attention of further executives, then you're really going to be setting yourself up for failure.

Others recognized that individual initiative and "self-awareness" played an important role but was not the only driver. As one leader explained,

> I think part of that is the training the Navy gave me and exposing me to the right training opportunities and the right job. And a lot of it had to do with having the right mentors that made sure they advocated for me for when the jobs became available. . . . On top of all that, I think, there's probably a baseline of self-awareness and self-study that an individual has to have to begin with so that they can recognize opportunities for that kind of growth within themselves. And I don't know where that comes from. I don't know how I got that, you know? I just know it was there before all this started.

Finally, another leader noted that once in command, "It's basically self-development."

How to Incentivize

Many respondents (five) described promotion criteria and the desire to get promoted as primary incentives for individuals to seek out certain job assignments and development opportunities. Some characterized this as "checking off" or "ticking" the right boxes.

A few leaders were very clear about these motivational effects. One commander explained,

> What the majority of . . . people in the medical profession are concerned with is simply promotion. Most of them really have no desire to be the commanding officer or the executive officer or the king of anything or the queen of anything. But they do want to get promoted, because promotion—not only is it a sign of recognition and some prestige to be promoted, but it comes with pay benefits. And it comes with some other accoutrements. And you can get a better parking spot and that kind of stuff.

This leader went on to explain that nurses are well aware that they need a graduate degree to get promoted from O-5 to O-6 and that, unless they take an administrative position when they reach the O-4 level, "you're never going to get promoted." Others linked their own decision to seek education and assignments to promotion incentives. For example, one commander, a practitioner, sought out the administrative side of the house to become more competitive and get promoted: It was "getting that check in the box." The commander similarly identified promotion as the rationale for attending war college and obtaining an advanced degree:

> Nobody told me I had to take it or it was a requirement, but I knew that it would benefit my career and promotion opportunities if I had taken those classes. . . . And it doesn't say that, you know, in order to be promoted for O-6, you need to complete the following courses or the JPME that the Army and the Air Force

people have. Navy doesn't have any of that. And it's sort of word by mouth, and you may want to consider taking this, or you may want to consider taking that or doing this in order to make yourself more competitive. I'm trying to stand out of the bunch of grapes and say, "Hey, you know, I'm the bigger, plumper one here, because I've done this and this."

Several other leaders noted that the Surgeon General of Navy Medicine declared that he would not select anyone to be an MTF commander unless they had operational experience, and, as a result, "a flurry of people that hadn't had it . . . ran over to do it."

Two leaders mentioned that nurses must maintain clinical skills and competence to retain their credentials.

This credentialing requirement served as an incentive for individuals to perform a certain number of clinical hours each year or attend certain courses that fulfilled this requirement (e.g., advanced cardiac life support).

Related to the issue of retention, several leaders identified the Navy's inability to offer financial incentives as a constraint on selecting and developing leaders.

According to one respondent, "You can't go out and recruit; you can't offer bonuses and bring in who you want to bring in. You can't filter your own team . . . so you have to sort of work with the cards you're dealt."

Outcome

Many respondents (eight) noted that current Navy medical leaders lacked skills related to business, finance, and management.

When asked whether there were any areas in which current leaders were not adequately prepared, many respondents cited a lack of business and management skills. Others offered this observation unsolicited when discussing leadership more generally. For example, one respondent believed that clinical leaders needed a better understanding of the administrative side of the house (and the converse as well, that administrators needed a better appreciation for the clinical side of the house):

The clinical side often is completely clueless as to anything dealing with administration. For example, dealing with credentials, and privileging, and quality counsel, and quality issues the hospital administrator frequently doesn't understand. What all that means or why it's important is because we're interested in things being on time, and lined up straight, and the flight getting up, and that sort of thing. On the clinical side, they seem to have really no idea about IT systems, and why can't we do this, and the budgeting, and the difference between appropriations, what's the difference between operation and maintenance, and other procurement, and things that administration kind of takes for granted. So I think we need to put more emphasis on teaching the clinical side about how administration works, and we need to put more emphasis on the administrators, teaching them how the clinical side works.

Other respondents similarly attributed this weakness to clinical leaders or leaders with medical backgrounds. One respondent noted that specialists often lacked competence in business and finance, adding that "most of them don't even take care of it at home." Three leaders highlighted weaknesses with regard to the soft skills of managing and mentoring people. A few other respondents were more specific about particular deficit areas, such as leading organizations that include military, civilian, and contract workers.

Other reported areas of weakness included the following:

- *Humanitarian civil assistance and maritime strategy:* Several people working for one respondent were trying to learn how to perform disaster relief, nation building, partnership building, and related activities. The respondent was trying to learn how to lead them in these efforts.
- *Clinical skills:* One respondent noted that clinical skills suffer when one takes on a leadership position. This was a major concern because the lack of postcommand opportunities meant a possible return to clinical work at the end of the respondent's CO tour: "It's scary thinking of going back to any job that would put me in a full-time clinician billet."

Advice for Improving Leader Development

Three respondents urged for significant changes in the system and new thinking with regard to career paths.

One wanted the Navy to "break out of the mold," move away from the "lock-step career path," and also create more diversity among leaders. Another wanted the Navy to "move beyond rank":

I would say give responsibility earlier on, where possible. I think we should look beyond the rank boundaries and if we identify a person, a lieutenant who's capable of doing an O-4 or an O-5 job, that may or may not do it better than an O-4 or an O-5, we should look at that. We do tend at times to be very rank-conscious and reticent to step outside of that structure and say, "Okay, I'm going to name this O-3 to be the division head over these O-4s because I think they're a better performer and I think they can do the job more efficiently than the O-4s." I would say that rank is there for a reason, but it shouldn't be held up as the end-all of everything.

A third wanted to formalize training programs and requirements for getting into executive medicine and to create greater transparency regarding career paths to leadership.

Two respondents argued that leader training and development needed to occur earlier in one's career.

"Give people the tools early on and not later," advised one leader. The other similarly believed that providing coursework prior to assignments would help leaders know what is expected of them.

Some leaders had specific suggestions for improving the content of training.

One felt strongly that there was a need to develop training on how to supervise contract, civilian, and military leaders working together in an MTF. Another emphasized the need for greater preparation for business management: "I think we need to put more emphasis on teaching the clinical side about how administration works, and we need to put more emphasis on the administrators, teaching them how the clinical side works."

Other recommendations included the following:

- Give opportunities to leaders to start as COs in small facilities and then move to larger facilities.
- Work on the postcommand career track and opportunities for leaders.
- Create more opportunities for civilian leadership development.
- Work on retention issues: Attend to work-life balance issues to attract and retain individuals, potential leaders, and leaders.

Findings from Interviews with Air Force Health Professions Officers

The information in Appendixes C through E provided the input for the cross-case analysis reported in Chapter Four.

This appendix presents the findings drawn from our interviews with Air Force officers. This analysis draws primarily on 2008 interviews with respondents who were primarily MTF commanders. We also used material from the 2007 interviews, although they used a somewhat different protocol; not all were transcribed, many were less comprehensive, and few were from interviewees with individuals at the same MTF, meaning that not all were MTF commanders. We refer to all respondents in a gender-neutral way to ensure anonymity, but our sample included men and women. As a reminder, at the beginning of the interviews, respondents were informed that when we asked about leader competencies and development, we meant executive-level health professions officers, such as the commander of an MTF, chief medical officer, chief nurse, and others at that level.

Context, Organizational Environment, and Organizational Leader Expectations

Context and Organizational Environment
Many respondents (six) directly described the medical community reporting to the line community as influencing expectations for executive-level health professions officers.

Unlike the Army and the Navy, the Air Force medical community "works under the line," while the path from the MC to the Surgeon General is "fuzzy." Respondents described how this structure resulted in a different way of looking at qualifications of health care professionals, with more of a focus on military leadership than clinical expertise. As one respondent noted,

> I actually work for the wing commander, who is a nonmedical person. And so when they look to select leaders, they aren't necessarily selecting the good medical

person. They are looking for the well-rounded military leader who can deal with many things; because I serve in a senior leadership role for the entire installation based on being on his senior staff.

Respondents thought that this system was appropriate and beneficial. For instance, two respondents noted,

I'm another tool for our senior commanders to get the mission done. So I think that the guys who are ultimately responsible for getting the mission done should be the pickers of the leaders underneath them.

We report to the line community. I like that. And I think most of us do, because we feel very firm attachment to the mission that we're trying to do as a unit.

One respondent stated that this command structure had implications during joint or integrated missions with the other services:

And that's currently what we find most of the time as we're trying to now integrate services, is we just view things differently. Our frames of reference are different. And I think, too, what makes it different, especially for the Air Force, is that we work for the line of the Air Force. My boss . . . works for a line commander, a four-star general. So we are accountable to the line for everything we do. And in the Army and the Navy, they work within a medical command, which is very different.

Related to this, a couple of respondents noted that the process for and meaning of promotion and rank differed in the medical and line communities. One respondent described how rank equates to leadership for the line community, but not necessarily for the MC and DC:

The Medical Corps and Dental Corps tend to use promotion opportunity as a retention and recruiting tool. And so we have a lot of full colonels that are not necessarily good leaders. They're great clinicians, and that's what we're paying them for, and that's what we want to keep them for. But they're not necessarily good leaders. On the line side, the line cannot understand how you can have so many O-6s who aren't leaders. But that really is the distinction on the line side. It truly is a pyramid. Within the medics, we admittedly promote more than we should if it is based solely on leadership. So rank and leadership does not always correlate.

One respondent described how this situation could lead to a poor perception of the medical force by the line:

Because [of] our system, physicians don't do professional military education until they are lieutenant colonels. So the first professional military education they do, that benefits them for their progression, is the last one that most of the rest of us do. And because of the lack of emphasis on development as a military leader, the medical force often enjoys a very stereotypically negative stance in the eyes of line leadership. You know, we're not real officers. We're just medics. You hear that far too often—most often not deserved, sometimes very clearly deserved.

Respondents described the system of selection and competition for rank, and some described differences among corps in terms of leadership positions.

All respondents noted that there was competition for rank within corps but not across corps; a couple of respondents described this as being "best in breed" rather than "best in show." A few respondents thought that the system had a direct influence on the type of leaders selected (see the section "Outcome," later in this appendix).

In addition, respondents discussed the leadership opportunities available to individuals in different corps. Several respondents noted that command of bedded facilities was reserved for physicians. One respondent noted that this practice differed from that in the civilian community and felt that this decision had an impact on retention of MSC officers:

And while in the civilian medicine, obviously, you find health care administrators at the pinnacle of leadership, the Medical Service Corps does not have those opportunities. And even in the last five years, one of the things that demoralized a bunch of us was the decision by the Surgeon General that only physicians can command bedded facilities. Many people made a decision about the terminus of their career based on that decision. Friends of mine left in the last few years because of that.

Another respondent perceived the following rationale for that decision:

The Air Force, in the last several years, has taken a position that physicians, if possible, should command at hospitals because that's the way they can remain clinically current. So, in other words, a surgeon cannot maintain his or her privileges and remain clinically competent and able to deploy if they're commanding a clinic or a small hospital that does not do surgery.

One former BSC officer (who switched corps) described the lack of leadership opportunities in the BSC:

There were two big factors that were very clear to me, even as a very junior officer, and that was the Biomedical Science Corps is essentially a hodgepodge of 16 or 17 specialties, not necessarily aggregated because they go together, but they just seem to be everybody else. And that affects the cohesion and how the corps at a corporate level works. And that certainly cascades down. You even feel that as a Biomedical Science Corps officer, as a very junior officer, that somehow it just seems to be different than the other corps, and it's kind of a thrown-together caste.

At the time, clearly, the Medical Service Corps had opportunities for promotion and advancement that far exceeded what I felt the Biomedical Science Corps was going to offer me. And I think that still is a perception, though it's gotten better.

Leader Expectations

Many respondents (seven) mentioned experience as an important criterion for leaders—particularly experience in a broad set of assignments.

Respondents described the need to spend time in multiple commands to obtain broad experiences and to gain experience outside of one's core competency, and highlighted career progression through multiple commands. As one respondent noted, "So to really develop somebody's skill set and an understanding of our system, they really need to be moving around and understanding why MacDill is different from Altus, and it's different from Grand Forks and Yokota in Japan." Another respondent described how these multiple positions helped leaders gain an understanding of how the medical community contributes to the Air Force's overall mission:

> So by the time I was a major, I'd already been in the United States, and I'd been in the Pacific Forces, and then I'd been in Europe. And then I come back, and then I go to do a residency. And then I go back, and then I go into Air Combat Command, and then I go back to Europe. And then I come back to the States, and I go to senior service school. And then I go to a medical center; I go to Air Education and Training Command. And then I go to the Air Force Academy. And then I go to a combatant command. So you can see, I think a leader that gets a broad perspective of multiple major commands, also, and the multiple positions on the globe, I think contributes, again, to understanding what our mission is in the United States Air Force.

Soft leadership skills, including communication skills, were also seen as necessary by many leaders (seven).

Many respondents considered "interpersonal skills" or "people skills" important for military medical leaders. A few respondents described the need for leaders to take care of their people and to develop them, acting like a "good parent." Others described how good leaders create receptive, positive climates that "people can grow in."

Some respondents (five) noted the value of communication skills. These leaders cited the importance of being able to communicate vision and mission objectives. As one leader explained, "Interpersonal skills have been key . . . because a lot of it is not what you do individually but how well you inspire and you influence others to achieve those organizational objectives." Another went as far as to say, "I think the single greatest determinant of a leader, military or civilian, is their ability to communicate verbally and in writing."

One described how these soft skills were key to motivating people to meet objectives:

> You need strong communication and people skills. I think what we do is manage a very diverse group of experts, from some specially trained surgeons to house-keeping staff. And what we're really about is really kind of a resource-constrained environment, keeping them to task, focused on the mission, and understanding the mission and their contribution, so they can feel fulfilled in what they're doing in their jobs day in and day out.

Many respondents (six) described the need for systems thinking, strategic planning, and an understanding of the larger organizational context.

Some respondents described excellent leaders as possessing a "global perspective," being systems thinkers, and "understanding the Air Force system" and the medical community's "role in the organization." Reflecting the unique Air Force structure, a couple of respondents directly noted the importance of understanding the line and the medical perspective. According to one,

> I think a line leader is going to be somebody that has come up in the system and understands the system and has a good grasp of big picture. And a medical leader, I think, is pretty much the same thing: Come[s] up through the system, under-stands the big picture, has the orientation on the mission of the Air Force to fly, fight, and win, and balances that against the needs of the beneficiary population.

Another respondent described how high-potentials see the larger health care system and overall strategy:

> I think the high-potential officers are ones that get out of their comfort zone, so to speak—out of their specialty—and they start putting the pieces of the larger health care puzzle together. And they start to become better systems thinkers, better strategists, better planners.

Some respondents (five) described executive skills or business skills as important to leadership and command of medical facilities. These leaders described the need for finance, logistics, and general business skills needed to effectively lead and manage an MTF. However, one respondent thought that leaders did not need to be experts in some of these areas (e.g., budgeting); rather, they needed to know what questions to ask to make the decisions.

Respondents agreed that medical leaders needed to have excelled in their clinical field; how-ever, opinions were mixed on whether leaders needed to retain those clinical skills.

While a few interviewees described trying to retain their clinical skills, others thought that it was impractical for senior leaders to continue practicing. One respondent argued what was important was clinical credibility, not simply operating in the clinics:

> A senior leader's probably not going to be in the clinics. But I have to have come from that world. I have had to come from that world. So I would argue that the investment in a senior leader who has been there, who can empathize with— doesn't matter whether you're a nurse, or a public health officer, or a lab officer, or a doc—but who can empathize and understand the world, [is the result of] credibility.

One interviewee described a similar situation for line pilots: "You don't have your hand on the stick once they make two-star." Another respondent spoke of the need to prioritize leadership over clinical skills:

> From my level, what I would say is it's more important to understand what the clinicians at the bedside are doing than it is to be perfecting my clinical skills. I mean, if I know I'm in the bucket, and I'm going to deploy in a clinical position, yeah, it's absolutely incumbent on me to go out and get my clinical skills refreshed. But on a day-to-day basis, where I am in the organization, it's my job to know more about what is working well and what isn't working well, what are the issues at the clinical level, so that I at the executive table can represent nursing needs adequately and appropriately. I think you have to temper that, but in my role, because it's strategic based, I have to be able to articulate the needs of this huge nursing force, and if I spend too much time concentrating on my own skills, then I lose visibility. So I can't compartmentalize myself. It's a delicate balance.

Although a few respondents discussed JMESP competencies, no one spoke of them as being relevant or used as measures of leader competency.

As one leader put it, JMESP "is not really utilized that well in picking or developing leaders."

Most respondents attested to the value of leaders understanding how the other services operate, particularly since the Air Force operates in more joint situations, but leaders were more mixed in their views about mandatory joint qualifications.

In most interviews, we asked respondents their opinions about the extent to which executive leaders needed joint experience and education and whether they believed these requirements should be mandatory. In discussing "joint," most referred to interoperability, integration, and interdependence with other services rather than formal joint billets. One respondent discussed the different conceptions of joint directly:

Joint is a word that is thrown around cavalierly and remains not defined. There are some who would say joint means green. There are some [to whom] joint means interoperable, and there are some [to whom] joint means interchangeable. All of those are different.

While only two respondents thought that joint experience should be mandatory for making general, many thought that joint experiences were of growing importance. One described them as "critical" and "essential." A couple of respondents stated that joint concepts were increasingly common due to the wars. As one respondent noted,

> We fight joint. We deploy and set up joint operations. I'm going to Afghanistan in a couple months. I'm going to be the team leader of a joint medical team, plus coalition, plus [nongovernmental agencies], plus the interagency.

Other factors important for high-quality medical leaders, mentioned by a few respondents, included qualities such as vision, flexibility, decisionmaking ability, ability to manage change, and ability to manage competing goals and priorities.

Approach to Leader Development

Although our interview protocols and questions emphasized leader development—how and when individuals are identified for leader development opportunities and the specific opportunities provided—respondents often answered by describing who was selected as a leader and when. This likely had to do with how the services define leadership development: Much depends on experience (i.e., giving someone the opportunity to lead and gain on-the-job experience to develop them as a leader). As a result, the following themes blend both areas: identifying leaders and identifying individuals for leader development.

Most respondents considered the Air Force to have a reasonable and well-defined system in place for leader development that included the flight paths and development teams.

Almost all referred to the flight path that provides an overview of the career trajectories for officer by corps. One respondent explained,

> Yes, we have a career path that is laid out in kind of a pyramidal shape that is published to everybody in our career field, Medical Service Corps, that shows the different things that should be accomplished along the way as you go toward the top of the pyramid, the jobs. . . . I think it's pretty well laid out, what's expected.

Several respondents also mentioned development teams as the formal process for managing careers. One respondent described the development team process in the DC:

> Now in the dental world, we actually get together on a regular basis and go, "Let's look at all the lieutenant colonels," and we vector them on leadership, academics, or clinical, and this is true of all the corps. And we say, "This person is really strong as a teacher, then let's not put him in as a commander; let's let him run a program and teach people." Or, "This person is really good as a clinician, but he doesn't want to run." . . . So we actually—all five of the corps now—pretty much keep lists not for jobs, but for natures of skills. And [we] say, "This guy is going this way, and this guy is going that way, and this guy is going that way."

Another leader described the creation of the Air Force's leadership development system and framework:

> Three to four years ago, we developed what we call the AFMS [Air Force Medical Service] flight path on the air staff. There were a couple of guiding principles in this development, and this flight path is what we are now executing right now. The guiding principles were basically that we did want to develop career paths or career pyramids that we would be able to identify people with. We developed development teams along corps lines that would select folks not in a determinative fashion but more a suggestive fashion, who are most competent, most qualified to enter leader tracks, academic tracks, or pure clinical tracks. That development team incorporates their desires as well as the opinions of senior leaders in that at [the time of] determination.

Most respondents were positive about this formal process, and only one person thought that the Air Force did not do a good enough job of differentiating people and figuring out where they should fit in the organization.

A common theme throughout the interviews was that the way to develop people is to identify high-potentials and give them special opportunities (through command and education) to grow, prove themselves, and develop.

All respondents thought that it was high-potentials who were developed, and some described how these individuals were groomed and watched. (This point is discussed in greater detail in the discussion of assignments and training in the section "How to Develop," later in this appendix.) Respondents described a process by which high-potentials are identified and given bigger jobs, commands, and specialized training.

> In general, the high-potential ones are given leadership positions very early in rank, lieutenant even, captain. And once we identify the ones that we feel have true potential, we push them to bigger jobs, bigger leadership jobs, even at the intermediate command or the major command level. And we identify them for special

training programs, whether it's education with industry, or [to] get another graduate degree. I think the Medical Service Corps is pretty good at identifying the ones
that we think have high potential and specifically targeting them for training or
job opportunities that will build on their strengths.

One respondent described this as the Air Force identifying "special people" and
giving them "special opportunities." This person thought that the Air Force should
identify people as early as possible, develop them, and treat them according to their
potential:

> On the medical side of the house, I think we need to try to identify them early,
> and obviously it's a fairly big pool when they're captains, lieutenants, and it kind of
> shrinks as you go up, but one of the things is that we need to realize that we have
> some special people, and we need to treat them specially. And if you treat every-
> one the same, then what you end up with is a very mediocre product, because you
> treated your dirt bags the same way you treated your superstar. And like in pro
> football, if you paid your star quarterback the same thing that you paid your water
> boy, you would not have a very good quarterback, but you might have a very good
> water boy, but nobody would care, and you would lose games. And so, I think we
> have to identify those people, and have special things for them.

How to Select

Formal Means. Respondents identified formal evaluations as important, but some
questioned their consistency.

Respondents described the importance of evaluations in the leader identification process.

Several (eight) respondents described getting a below-the-zone promotion and
"getting ranked" on evaluations as the indicator that someone is a high-potential.
Respondents tended to acknowledge that evaluations were inflated. One respondent
said, "I joke the worst thing you can ever give someone is an honestly fair evaluation,
because without the inflation, they would be at the bottom of the barrel."

Nonetheless, respondents tended to believe that the evaluations did allow for the
identification of high-potential leaders due to the evaluators' use of a ranking system,
such as indicating that a given person is number one of 20 nurses. Ranking was seen as
a powerful indicator and a clear message to promotion boards. One respondent shared
a story of the power of this message:

> One of my old bosses told me about a promotion board he was sitting on, and on
> the thing it said, "Number 13 of 12 such and such," and they thought it was a
> typo, they thought it was probably number three of 12, so they called the writer
> and said, "What did you mean here? Was this a typo?" And he said, "Nope, that's
> exactly what I meant." And so the message is very clear, just from that stratifica-

tion. If you're sitting on a promotion board, you do not need to read any other words on that thing.

However, two individuals noted that the use of evaluations could be problematic if the rater doesn't possess good writing skills. One said that "careers can be ruined" because of this failure.

Another respondent described how the most senior leaders were selected by examining the candidates' entire profiles.

> I think it's usually a 1-to-10 scoring factor, and we talk about, you know, just the things that I've already mentioned. Have they completed their professional military education? Are they certified in a clinical area? What do their [officer performance reports] look like? Have they been stratified? That's huge. I mean, within their organization, has their senior rater said, "Out of a hundred nurses, this is number two"? We look at those kinds of things, and that's how we weight the record. So, it's a composite of all those factors. Not only have they completed their professional military education, but did they do it in residence? Because that's always a huge discriminator, because to go to do PME in residence is a big thing, because there is not a lot of opportunity within the Nurse Corps to do that, so that always is going to have additional weight.

Another individual noted that performance during emergency circumstances could influence how candidates rise to the top through evaluations and promotion boards.

> If something happens on your watch, and that's key, if something happens on your watch, you either perform or you don't. You either perform or you don't. It's that simple. And then, so if you got three or four guys that are all about the same level of potential, and if something happens on one . . . person's watch, and it goes well, that separates you from the pack.

Informal Means. Networking was mentioned as a key component of selection.

A few other respondents described a parallel informal system that influenced the identification of leaders as well.

One respondent described the informal factors at work:

> I also think that there's also the networking factor, and the cultural factor, and the timing factor for a lot of high-potential officers and opportunities that are out there. And to some degree, I think the fast burners—the folks that get out there and make the contribution, and do their thing—they get identified early. And then that's where the informal system kicks in.

Another respondent thought that the informal system was particularly important in determining who was assigned the most senior jobs, explaining that these assignments were based on reputation, separate from evaluation reports:

> And then, of course, when the senior leadership gets together . . . for the big assignments . . . we all know each other's reputations. And so we either respect each other's opinions or we don't. And so when we're looking at folks to fill the senior-level positions—and say especially on the staffs, not the squadron commanders, or not the group commanders, but the staff—you say, "Hey, this'll be a great guy. Did a great job for us over here at [Pacific Air Forces]. I think he'd do a great job on the Air Staff." So there's a lot of exchange of information that goes on, yes, at the senior level.

How to Develop

Job Assignments and Experiences. Respondents saw value in the Air Force's career paths and in joint positions, though they disagreed that the latter should be mandatory.

Almost all respondents described career progression on the route to flag officer as providing a range of experiences and command roles that progressively increased in responsibility.

One respondent explained how that progression built various experiences and increasingly broad views of the system for future generals:

> You [work] your way up. And so at each level, you branch out. . . . In other words, at some point, especially when you become a squadron commander, you're no longer just thinking about your flight surgeon's office. You're thinking about aerospace medicine, you're thinking about public health, you're thinking about biomedical engineering, you're thinking about health promotions. . . . When you go to the next level, of course, when you're a medical group commander, assuming that you took time to learn what the squadrons did while you were a squadron commander, then you're a better medical group commander. . . . So I think it's experience, it's exposure. I think you need to move, and you have leadership at all different levels.

Some respondents thought that this on-the-job training was the best way to train leaders. One leader said,

> The best way to learn anything is by doing it. So, by doing it, I've learned so much more than I would ever have learned in any textbook or course or discussions. It's the Air Force's way of rounding out folks and making sure they've got everything.

While many leaders considered joint experiences to be beneficial, only a few thought they should be mandatory.

Many leaders noted the limited supply of these joint positions. As one leader explained,

> For the experience in the joint arena, it presents a challenge because of the very limited number of positions that give you that full joint experience and joint flavor. I've been fortunate to be able to be in the joint environment, and I was also very fortunate to have joint education behind me that helped prepare me for the role.

One leader argued that the Air Force needed a certain number of the highest-level leaders to have this experience:

> Again, like I said, it's not necessary that all our general officers have joint experience. . . . But I think you need a certain number of us . . . in the joint job, because you need to have that perspective also at the senior leadership position. I call them the cabinet. But you need to have somebody on that cabinet, one or two or three of them, that have what I call joint experience. It would be nice if we all had it, but we don't all have it, I don't think, because we don't have the opportunity.

Two respondents described experiences in fellowships and residencies as a method of developing future leaders.

Respondents described specific programs:

> You can do a readiness fellowship, for instance, at the Air Combat Command. I mean, there's several fellowships out there, and we're always trying to identify those opportunities where we could offer fellowships to basically develop future leaders.

> One program I hadn't mentioned that has been very beneficial to identify high-performing leaders early is the Air Force intern program, and that is a way of identifying captains and getting them into various positions at the Pentagon or the Air Staff to expose them early in their career to some of the senior leadership decisions, strategic and operational planning, and that is a very good foundation for our more junior-grade officers to continue pursuing professional military education, various career tracks.

Education and Training. Respondents cited a range of training and education opportunities for high-potential officers, especially at the war colleges.

Respondents described a number of education opportunities provided to officers as they progressed through the leadership track.

Almost everyone described formal education and training received for certain positions at the squadron command and group command. Others mentioned obtaining graduate degrees under Air Force fellowships. One leader described the progression of education and training for MSC officers:

> Yeah, we start off with a three-month course when they first come in called Health Services Administration for all new MSC officers. They go through a three-month course which teaches them pretty much how the Air Force approaches health care administration. There's kind of a practical portion to that course as well as some classroom, didactic time. Then, we develop some people with internships in certain fields, like logistics. We start them off with an internship for about ten months, then they go off and take a staff position someplace in a hospital or clinic. But then, down the road, we also have fellowships that we offer, usually at the senior captain or major level, where they are given a fellowship to work somewhere . . . you know, a staff position someplace, maybe Air Staff or major command. In some cases, they are also at an area hospital level. We have a fellowship, for example, in medical readiness, and they have a chance to work in that function for ten months. We also do education with industry. And we send people off for master's degrees, too, usually at the lieutenant and junior captain level. And, of course, the PME that we talked about earlier is factored in for Medical Service Corps officers.

All respondents described PME opportunities offered to leaders, including the Air War College and National War College.

Attending the war colleges in residence was described as prestigious and a marker for potentially making general. As one respondent noted, "Officers who go to those courses are destined to higher levels of responsibility."

Respondents considered attending PME in residence far more beneficial than completing via correspondence. War college by correspondence was considered something that "checked a box." A couple of respondents who completed these programs via correspondence found the content to be too focused on the line: "It's geopolitics, and it's joint warfare and it's warfighting thinking, if you will, and it's not, 'Can you run a hospital?'"

In contrast, many respondents found these PME opportunities very valuable, particularly for those who attended in residence. One officer remarked,

> I was very fortunate to go to our three PME schools in the Air Force: Squadron Officer School in residence, Air Command and Staff College in residence, and Air War College in residence. They have been invaluable, not only to my role as a commander, but also in my work here at Joint Forces Command.

One officer described the skills addressed at war college as "essential" to leader development, in part because of the medical community's direct relationship to the line:

In the Air Force, [war colleges are] essential. Air Force medical leaders have to understand our mission, and that's the expectation of the Air Force line leadership. . . . They're going to expect for their medical leaders to either know the answer, or be able to find the answer—or be able to find the person who can find the answer.

Another leader focused on the need to develop as both a military officer and a medical officer:

I think that the way the Air Force approaches PME, which is all I'm familiar with—I've only gone to Air Force PME or taken it in my career—I think the way the Air Force approaches it does give the right approach, I guess. I have heard people in the medical field say that they think it's too line-centric and so forth, that there's not enough medical in there to teach the line what we're about and so forth, and they feel left out in some cases. I guess in my opinion, Air Force PME gives a good, broad picture of what we should be learning about. It's really a course to learn about how to be a military officer more than it is how to be a medical professional, a communications professional, a pilot, what have you. It's above career fields and it's [aimed] more at actually what an officer needs to be educated on, I guess, as part of being a professional officer. So, I think the Air Force does that pretty well, and the criticism of some saying that it's not really applicable to medical people, . . . I wouldn't agree with that, I guess. I think medical officers do need to understand the entire Air Force picture, and PME is one of the best ways to get that.

However, when asked whether medical leaders should receive additional slots to allow more to attend in residence, almost no one agreed with such a policy. As one officer noted,

Oh, it would be beneficial to the medics, but it would be detrimental to the line because you only have two other spots, so I would leave it like it is.

Several respondents described the Interagency Institute for Federal Health Care Executives at George Washington University. All respondents who attended this program found it beneficial because it focused on health care and provided exposure to interagency perspectives. As one respondent said,

That is interesting, because what they do is you get exposed to both of those, both medical executive skills and also interagency. But interagency, you learn [that] there's not only a DoD.

Another respondent described the benefit of the global perspective offered by the National War College and the Interagency Institute for Federal Health Care Executives:

It gives you an opportunity to understand that there are other folks out there, all potentially . . . could be your allies, or potentially vying for the same resources. That was one of the things, when I was at U.S. Central Command. In order for us to win this global war on terrorism, I would argue that the DoD is probably 15 percent of the solution. The other 85 percent of that is the interagency. Yes. And I understood that a little bit better before I got there because of, again, having the exposure to some of these other interagencies: one through the National War College, which is, again—you remember—that's not only Army, Navy, Air Force, Marine Corps, but that's also interagency—CIA, FBI, State Department. I remember a guy that was one of my homeroom mates, so to speak, in our homeroom. The guy sitting to my right was going off to be the deputy in x. So I spent a lot of time talking to him about the State Department. So I understood that, and then again, those conversations offline at the National War College and also Interagency Institute. But understanding that, I felt maybe a little bit more knowledgeable in understanding what it's going to take to do what we do during my [U.S. Central Command] assignment. Yes, absolutely.

Several respondents identified areas in which more education might be needed, including writing skills and formalized business training, especially in budgeting and manpower.

Furthermore, one respondent thought that the education opportunities provided to medical leaders were "inadequate in preparing people to manage a health care system."

Mentoring. Respondents saw informal mentoring arrangements as more valuable than the Air Force's formal mentoring program.

While several people mentioned that the Air Force has a formal mentoring system, all described the informal system, and only one person discussed the formal system.

The formal system was described as a failure that was no longer followed:

We tried a formal mentoring program a few years ago where people signed up on the computer and selected who their mentor was and all that. And it was just a flop because it was way too formal; it was way too stilted and it doesn't work.

Respondents tended to value "natural" mentorships over a formal mentor system. As one leader explained,

A natural mentorship versus the kinds you sometimes see in organizations trying to force mentorships, which in my opinion is not the way we should mentor people. . . . Again, in my opinion, mentorship is kind of a natural thing that happens between two people.

Almost all respondents described mentoring or being mentored.

Mentor relationships were initiated from both the top and the bottom. Some respondents described reaching out to a specific senior officer based on a common interest, while others talked about looking for young officers to mentor and the desire to "find your replacement." Many described the importance of "mentoring the next generation of leaders." One respondent explained,

> Each of us in more senior positions, I think, has a 3×5 card where we've written down or sketched out the dozen or so folks that we have under our wing, so to speak . . . folks that come to us for advice. That's my favorite part of the job, quite frankly: the young physicians and enlisted members of the team—physicians, nonphysicians, and enlisted members of the team—that come to me for advice. I do, I sit down with each one of them. We map out their career on a timeline, we go over their options and desires, and I go over with them . . . next steps and what the expectations are. . . . But it's an informal approach. It's very individual. I think that, again, that's an innate part of being an Air Force medical leader is that each of us takes pride in growing those folks who will take our place.

This leader also described giving mentees opportunities to experience greater command levels on a temporary basis:

> And, as I'm selecting people within my group or within my wing for leadership positions, I will very deliberately pull people out and put them in temporary positions, at least, where I know they're out of their element, because I want to push them. I want to see how they can expand into that mission environment.

Respondents reiterated the importance of mentoring at all levels:

> I do think it's very important to capture opportunities and continue to, as a supervisor, develop our individuals who have that thirst, for growth, especially, and then also to seek professional development mentoring from those senior. And knowing the brick and mortar facility is great; knowing the joint operational environment is great. And just continue to be able to grow, develop, mentor, and continue to serve, I think, is all very important. I have to say, I've had great opportunities in my career and I've just been very fortunate to have mentors over the years to open and afford me those opportunities. I'm just very pleased to be able to share what I have learned and mentor some of the more junior officers developing today.

One respondent said that training was heavily dependent on mentorship, describing mentors as helping junior leaders understand where they are, where they needed to go, and how to get the required knowledge set.

Career Counseling. Unlike in the other two services, career counseling was cited as a formal feature of Air Force leader development.

Respondents described career counseling as a part of the formal development team process.

One respondent explained,

So this has only been within the last few years that I, as the corps chief, preside over a twice-a-year meeting where we bring together the, if you will, the chief of professional services. So, not the commander, but the kind of the most senior doc from all our major commands. Again, we do that differently than the Army. But so let's say there's, you know, seven or eight major commands and a few smaller ones. We bring them together. We get them in a room, and we say, "Okay, here's a list of all of your majors who have been promoted to lieutenant colonel, all of your lieutenant colonels, and all of your lieutenant colonels promoted to colonel." . . . And we send every one of them a letter that says, "Put in your request for your career, major, lieutenant colonel, colonel select, and then we'll tell you the vector we think you should be on." And so we will sit around a table. We will identify strengths and weaknesses, and then we'll give them feedback as to which way they should go. So it was using that kind of basic structure that we then sent out [feedback] to everybody, every lieutenant colonel select, lieutenant colonel, or colonel select, and said, "Are you interested in applying for these 20 slots? We've got funding for 20 slots. Are you interested?" And I think we had about 80 people apply. And so we whittled down to the 20, and then we're all going to have a competitive board at the same developmental team meeting to look at then how we select the five a year that I've secured funding for.

Another respondent said that people are emailed advice periodically (e.g., "Time for you to consider *x*.") by their development team.

Feedback. Feedback was primarily discussed under the development team process (see the previous discussion of career counseling). However, one individual described how performance reports, when done well, provided feedback to officers.

When I had my staff give me input for their performance reports, you know, tell me what you did this last year, I tell them to give it to me on a 10-scale, if you will; that if they think they're an 8, and I think they're a 2, we're going to have an opportunity to discuss. If they think they're an 8, and I think they're a 7, that's good. That means we're close. We have a similar perspective on how they're doing. And it serves as a form of feedback. So I think the [officer performance report] process is good, if done correctly. And not everyone does.

Self-Development. A few respondents described self-initiated development that they felt helped them develop as leaders. Respondents mentioned taking short courses in areas such as budget management or writing, attending conferences from civilian organizations, and maintaining certification through civilian accrediting bodies.

How to Incentivize

Several respondents noted that various "development opportunities" greatly affected promotion and that the incentive of looking good when coming before boards and being considered for selection drove officers to seek out educational opportunities and new positions.

A key example of this was advanced PME courses. A few respondents noted that some people attend Air University or Air War College, particularly by correspondence, only because it is a requirement for promotion. As one leader explained,

> So our guys whine about it, but they'll do it just because they want to make colonel, and those who don't do it really don't get promoted. I mean, it's a very real thing, but when you ask them, "Okay, so you did it?" they'll go, "Yeah, well, I had to. We'd never have done it if I didn't have to."

Outcome

Several respondents held very positive views about the skills and abilities of current medical leaders.

Current medical leaders were seen as high-quality personnel, and many respondents thought the Air Force's process did a good job of grooming high-potential candidates. In particular, one individual recognized the flight path and development teams for improving the process and leadership quality:

> I think we do a fairly good job of . . . defining the flight path in the different corps, so that we use your experience, we use your core competency, we get you some experience in the joint world and looking at other aspects and operations in our Air Force, and then bring them back to be the senior leaders. Personally, I think we're as healthy as we've ever been on it. Other folks don't agree with me, but I think it's a lot better than it was before, because it was rather random before.

However, some respondents expressed concerns about how the "best in breed" competition affected the quality of the outcome. Several thought that competition within corps resulted in suboptimal leadership choices. As one individual said, "The best people in a corps may not be the best people for the job." One leader was concerned that the process of board and command selection could lead to suboptimal positioning of people due to timing issues.

Advice for Improving Leader Development

Respondents offered ideas about how to expand the skills of upcoming leaders in the various corps.

Respondents thought that nurses could use more line mentorship for command roles. They also believed that MSC members could benefit from gaining a better clinical perspective, understanding patient needs and the time it takes to fulfill those needs, by spending time as patient advocates or by shadowing clinicians. They also stated that the DC would benefit from earlier exposure to experiences outside of that corps.

One individual thought that the Air Force should focus on retaining and developing for leadership roles the doctors who were doing something "different" in the Air Force from what they would be doing in the civilian word, because these individuals may be more committed to military service. That respondent suggested that the Air Force "focus more on retaining flight surgeons and less on pediatricians, OB/GYN."

A few respondents had advice with regard to education and training.

A few respondents felt that the Air Force should expand exposure to joint issues during training programs. Another thought that the services should coordinate to identify the best courses offered internally and in the civilian sector to address the 40 (now 39) JMESP competencies and to provide a certificate or master's degree upon completion of the set of experiences. This individual explained,

> To me, there are so many opportunities to develop competence and leadership. . . . What is needed is to pull those [education programs] all together: Army, Navy, Air Force, Marines, Georgetown University, you name it. Identify the best existing courses that answer the 40 competencies. . . . When the DoD has identified the best opportunities to fill their 40 competencies there's got to be a certificate and master's degree credit at the end of it. And that is so imminently doable. That would take . . . a triservice staff of about six or eight people that come together, identify what we're already doing. In other words, don't invent new courses, except maybe the joint medical officer's course. That might be a good thought. Bring them together, identify what we already have going on, figure out which one's best. What does the Air Force do, what does the Navy do, what does the Army do, what does the Coast Guard do that best prepares people to fill that square under the 40? And then award them academic credit and get them embarked on a lifelong journey to end up with a master's in medical management [or] an MBA.

A few respondents thought that the Air Force should move away from competition within corps and move back to competition across corps.

This view was certainly not shared by all, however. One respondent argued,

> I think we need to get away from this kind of careerist, "We need to push *x* number of whatever through the system so they have a promotion opportunity." I think we need to pay people what they're worth but not link it to leadership, which is what we do. And I think that's a mistake. . . . We don't need to set a quota. And that's true for every corps, whether it be Medical Service Corps officers [or others]. If we can't get ten a year that are going to fit the bill to be leaders at the group or whatever level, then we don't need to just pick the wrong ten and force them into positions they're not qualified for.

Two respondents suggested middle-of-the-road approaches. One respondent suggest making job assignments by corps "guidance" rather than a mandate or quota. In the same vein, another respondent thought it would be beneficial to have the option to give command positions to other corps. He noted,

> But then the problem there is that, depending on supply in any given year, you might not have the right mix, so the pendulum has now gone to where it is very prescriptive, and you have to occasionally go, "I didn't have enough candidates to do my share. You got more candidates in the nursing. Why don't we swap?" But we're not to that level yet. We're getting there.

Selected Examples of Leader Development Programs Implemented by Civilian Health Care Organizations

This appendix provides some examples of education and training programs implemented by civilian health care organizations as part of the leader development approaches described in Chapter Five.[1] The information presented here was current as of 2008.

Internal Development Opportunities Designed Specifically for Senior Executives

Kaiser Permanente has a five-week advanced leadership program that is described as a "watered-down MBA" that involves leaders in diverse roles from throughout the system who are being considered for high-level positions. The program involves simulations, reviews of business cases, and more didactic teaching on such topics as how to interact with the press. It is an expensive program but was seen as extremely valuable by the executive we interviewed.

HCA's COO Development Program is focused on training future COOs who are likely to become CEOs. It is a three- to five-year program and involves about 45 individuals per cohort (there are two classes per year). Participants are recruited from MHA and MBA programs as well as internally (there is a 50-50 external-internal split). Once accepted, a participant is assigned to a hospital in an administrative role (at the organization's expense, so it is free to the hospital). The participant is mentored by the hospital's CEO, receives targeted training, and ultimately is placed in a COO position when one opens up and the participant is deemed ready. The program follows an 80-10-10 model: 80 percent development through work on the job, 10 percent through mentoring, and 10 percent through structured learning at the corporation's office headquarters, organized around key competencies, such as physician relations, patient satisfaction, and strategic planning. Structured learning also includes cases and

---

[1] This information was taken from materials provided by the organizations or accessed through web and literature searches.

real projects, such as budgeting or capital asset planning and reporting back to the group.

HCA sponsors a similar program for nurses, focused on developing future CNOs. Although HCA puts forth a substantial investment for both programs, they are seen as not only a great growth and networking opportunity for participants, but also a valuable way of moving ideas and best practices around the organization.

Yale's New Haven Healthcare's Leadership Academy enrolls approximately 12 people at any one time and is described as focusing on "how to manage oneself." It starts with a self-assessment and 360-degree evaluation. The program meets three to four times per year in four- or five-day sessions off-site with external faculty. The program focuses on managing across functions, managing other managers, and influencing in a matrix environment. It also includes follow-on coaching to ensure application and transfer of knowledge.

The Mayo Clinic organizes a three- to four-day leader development program for senior leaders (e.g., department chairs) and their direct reports. It involves approximately 250 people and is organized around a topic of strategic importance to the clinic, such as safety or quality. The program also includes guest speakers (e.g., the CEO of IBM). The Mayo Clinic also sponsors a one-week course for high-potentials being groomed for leadership positions that focuses on personnel development, mentoring, finance, and system engineering.

The Cleveland Clinic sponsors "C-level tutorials" for high-potential leaders, who generally attend eight at a time. The sessions involve projects and generally provide participants with an opportunity to determine whether they are interested in taking on more administrative leadership. The Cleveland Clinic also nominates individuals to attend an academy program one day per week for six months. The program's curriculum focuses on marketing, finance, and personnel and includes visits from guest speakers from within the organization.

The Palo Alto Medical Foundation sends leaders to its parent company's Sutter Health Leadership Academy, modeled after a program run by General Electric. The foundation nominates eight people each year to participate for one year. On Fridays and Saturdays, physician leader-administrator pairs meet to learn about topics such as finance, negotiation, system design, and process flow and to participate in 360-degree reviews and psychological profiling.

Former executives at Virginia Mason and Trinity Health also described senior leader development programs that were team-based. At Trinity, the past leadership program involved six to eight participants who met three to four times a year for a week of intensive classes, education, and simulations. The program mixed individuals from large and small organizations belonging to the health system, as well as individuals with clinical and management backgrounds. Virginia Mason's past executive team professional development included approximately 25 participants in a series of three two-day events. The events generally started with a set curriculum, assessments to understand personal leadership or conflict styles, and the practice of certain skills (e.g., via role playing). Then, participants were given an assignment, such as a project in their department, and reported back on what they learned. One executive believed that these programs were very valuable:

> It's unique in a sense that many times you go off to a training course, and you get new ideas and things that [make you say], "Gosh, I wish everybody in leadership at Virginia Mason would know about this." . . . But rarely did they have the opportunity that everyone's learning the same thing at the same time and can have common language. I think they found it very valuable. They came to understand each other in ways that they had never had the opportunity to know each other before.

In addition to the specific examples noted here, several organizations sponsor retreats for top leaders, which serve as both a strategic planning activity for the organization and a development activity for individual leaders.

Internal Development Opportunities Designed Specifically for Clinical Leaders

One hospital sponsors a voluntary physician leader development program for approximately 25 community physicians (not employed by the hospital) to provide them with traditional leadership skills and education on health care issues from a hospital perspective. The program involves participants in a "capstone project," such as determining how to move patients through the system. Another hospital asked a university to develop a curriculum for its program, including case methods and experiential learning activities tied to the specific challenges of the hospital. In this new program, the department leaders will identify candidates and must promise time off for candidates to attend four times during a ten-month period, with each session lasting four full days. Participants will also engage in projects between the sessions. The program will focus on teamwork to help offset the "individualism" of physicians.

An article about the Cleveland Clinic described how its Leading in Health Care course evolved over time (Stoller, Berkowitz, and Bailin, 2007). More than 30 physicians were nominated to attend eight sessions, one per month, at an off-site retreat. The program focused on the development of a "business plan." Groups of four to six attendees were asked to identify a proposed innovation and develop a plan outlining its feasibility and implementation. In later years, nonphysician administrators were invited to serve as business plan "mentors." Research following up on the 49 plans submitted by participants over the years indicates that 30 (61 percent) had either been implemented or had "directly affected program implementation" (Stoller, Berkowitz, and Bailin, 2007, p. 240). For example, some plans for introducing new services or programs had been adopted (e.g., a "short stay" unit as an extension of the emergency room), while others helped spur process improvement (e.g., adoption of systemwide electronic medical records). The authors note that the activity provided "real-world context" to the application of concepts introduced in the coursework component of the program and also helped bond groups together to solve relevant problems. Additionally, the program created "a rich inventory of well-developed and critically evaluated ideas for institutional innovation and growth," and the implementation of plans represents "an important institutional return on the investment of developing and conducting the course" (Stoller, Berkowitz, and Bailin, 2007, p. 241).

Virginia Mason had developed a fellowship program in the Virginia Mason Production System for physicians with administrative roles. The fellowship involved intensive classroom learning, projects, and visits to Japan to study quality-management principles and concepts (e.g., flow).

External Professional Development and Educational Opportunities for Leaders

As noted in Chapter Five, it is common for organizations to sponsor external training or education for individuals with high potential.

Non-Degree-Granting External Opportunities

UK HealthCare of the University of Kentucky offers opportunities for those with potential to pursue development activities in areas in which they are interested. It was also in the midst of customizing a program for those being groomed to run the system's clinical ethics program. That candidate will be sent to various programs across the country. The system also planned to send some staff to Toyota for lean management training.

Beth Israel sends clinical leaders to an introductory course on health care management offered by the Harvard Business School. The organization's executive noted, however, that the only way potential leaders can put into practice what they learn without upsetting colleagues is to actually "do it" and apply it to their daily work.

Similarly, Vanderbilt sponsors individuals' attendance at Harvard's physician executive program and the Wharton School's programs for a month, paying all expenses. Moreover, many also earn a master's degree at Vanderbilt; the executive who we interviewed said that the arrangement created loyalty, among other things.

The University of Michigan Health System offers its Emerging Leader Program to directors and above, annually selecting about ten high-potential individuals for a week-long "global leadership training" course conducted by an external organization, the Global Leadership Institute. The program involves small workshops and speakers and draws from companies across the country; it is not specific to health care. Participants complete a leadership assessment before they attend and meet one on one with a coach while in the program to identify what they might do differently when they return to their institution. It was described as intense but highly rewarding for participants, who bond with one another during and after the program. Some participants are selected as a reward for strong performance; others may be selected because there is an area in which they need help.

OhioHealth senior leaders select individuals from the "high-potential" quadrant of the organization's talent grid and send them to the Center for Creative Learning's Leadership at the Peak program.

Henry Ford participates in LENS, sponsored by the NCHL. Its Advanced Leadership Development Program involves teams of executives from multiple organizations in weeklong sessions that provide coaching and support for using the NCHL leader competencies to address a major problem facing their organizations. Described as superior to programs offered by various universities, the program provides opportunities for participants to exchange ideas with others and develop skills. The Henry Ford executive explained,

> They also have an opportunity to bounce [ideas] off the other teams who are there working on their particular project and then sharing with each other what they've learned. For instance, we have a new community hospital that's under construction, which is kind of state-of-the-art from a people standpoint, from a patient standpoint, and from an employee standpoint. And one of the projects that we sent to the Advanced Leadership Development Program was for a team to lock themselves up for a week with the help of other teams to really kind of define what needed to be done in that organization.

Like Henry Ford, some organizations maximize the return on their investments in external professional development opportunities for select staff, which tend to be expensive, by asking participants to conduct projects for the organization when they return from the program or course. One respondent said that this was a good way to sustain the learning for participants and add value to the organization.

Degree-Granting External Opportunities

Many organizations pay the tuition for individuals to obtain advanced degrees. For example, the University of Wisconsin Hospitals and Clinics offer full scholarships to the executive MBA program at its affiliated university for future leaders at the manager or director level. The executive from this organization also gave an example of sponsoring someone in line for the chief information officer position to attend an executive MBA program and discussed the need to look at people individually. Similarly, Brigham and Women's Hospital pays people to take courses and attend degree-granting programs, such as the MPH in administration and management at Harvard. Several organizations reported annually sponsoring a group of physicians to obtain management degrees as a way to build up their skills to take on more leadership responsibilities. Many respondents also mentioned tuition-reimbursement programs and loan programs that apply to all staff.

Selected Senior Leader Development Programs Offered by the VA/VHA

This appendix describes selected additional programs used by the VA/VHA to develop its senior leaders according to the processes discussed in Chapter Six.[1] As mentioned earlier, the VHA is evaluating all its leadership programs, so they may change in the future.

VHA: Senior Executive Orientation

Originally designed for new facility directors, the program, which consists of four two-day seminars each year ("Leading for Results," "Leading People," "Relationships with Stakeholders," and "Effective Negotiation"), has been extended to newly appointed senior executives. A "coaching" component has also been added, using experienced directors as faculty and discussion leaders. The sessions include small-group discussions and other experiential formats and focus on practical issues faced by senior executives. Participants may begin the series at any point and make up missed sessions the following year.

VHA: Senior Management Conference

The VHA Senior Management Conference is offered on a periodic basis to current and emerging VHA leaders. The curriculum is built around current issues facing the organization and shares innovations in the delivery of health care to veterans. The conference provides a welcome opportunity for field leadership to gather with their VHACO colleagues and strengthen personal relationships and organizational bonds. Typically, the design of the conference offers a balance of plenary, breakout, and exhibit-type sessions.

---

[1] This information is taken from materials provided by the VHA.

VHA: Senior Executive Service Coaching Network

Recently implemented as a knowledge-transfer program, the intent of the network is "to support the transitioning and development of VHA senior executives as they transition into leadership positions that involve a significant change in the complexity or nature of their duties." The coaching network consists of current or recently retired senior executive service leaders who are or were in a leadership position of high complexity. The network provides leaders with the opportunity to meet regularly with a group of peers and an assigned coach to share experiences, challenges, and successes.

VA: Leadership VA

Leadership VA is a VA-wide program, unlike the others described here. It is part of an effort across the larger VA to help develop "an enterprise perspective." Leadership VA is a One VA–based executive development program that trains a minimum of 70 competitively selected participants per year. The program aims to expand participants' leadership skills, provide an opportunity to become acquainted with the VA's top leaders, and help participants develop a broader perspective on the internal and external forces that affect VA operations. The program also encourages the exchange of information and viewpoints to help broaden personal and professional perspectives.

One respondent described the program as follows:

> I'm a graduate of Leadership VA. . . . Leadership VA is a program that's been in place many years. It's an attempt to help an employee understand the bigger VA. Now the larger VA—I think we're the second-largest department after Defense. We have almost a quarter-million employees, or somewhere around there, in total. We have three divisions, as you know, VHA, VBA [Veterans Benefits Administration], and Cemetery. We tend to be in silos, and VHA doesn't know much about VBA or vice versa. This is a program where every year they take about 60 individuals and they try to bring on board 60 people to work from all three administrations and within the administration. So, if you will, you have a class mix and you spend four weeks together—four one-week sessions—in different experiential activities. Again, it's all about relationship-building. It finishes with an award ceremony with the Secretary for GS-13 and above. I graduated from that early in my career, and many of the people I met there are now [in] leadership today, and we'll still stay in contact. It's just a wonderful program from that end.

References

ACHE—*see* American College of Healthcare Executives.

ACPE—*see* American College of Physician Executives.

Air Force Instruction 36-2640, Executing Total Force Development, December 16, 2008.

Air Force Surgeon General, "Who We Are," web page, undated. As of May 26, 2010:
http://www.sg.af.mil/factsheets/factsheet.asp?id=8182

Air University, "Schools and Centers," web page, undated. As of May 26, 2010:
http://www.au.af.mil/au/schools.asp

AMEDD—*see* U.S. Army Medical Department.

American College of Healthcare Executives, "About ACHE," web page, undated. As of October 2007:
http://www.ache.org/aboutache.cfm

American College of Physician Executives, "The Story," web page, undated. As of October 2007:
http://www.acpe.org/Footer/AboutACPE.aspx

American Organization of Nurse Executives, "Welcome to AONE," web page, undated. As of May 26, 2010:
http://www.aone.org/aone/about/home.html

AONE—*see* American Organization of Nurse Executives.

Asch, Steven M., Elizabeth A. McGlynn, Mary M. Hogan, Rodney A. Hayward, Paul G. Shekelle, Lisa V. Rubenstein, Joan Keesey, John L. Adams, and Eve A. Kerr, "Comparison of Quality of Care for Patients in the Veterans Health Administration and Patients in a National Sample," *Annals of Internal Medicine*, Vol. 141, No. 12, December 21, 2004, pp. 938–945.

Baker, G. Ross, "Identifying and Assessing Competencies: A Strategy to Improve Healthcare Leadership," *Healthcare Papers*, Vol. 4, No. 1, July 2003, pp. 49–58.

Berry, Leonard L., and Kent D. Seltman, *Management Lessons from Mayo Clinic: Inside One of the World's Most Admired Service Organizations*, New York: McGraw-Hill, 2008.

Brannman, Shayne, Lauren Byrne, Senanu Asamoah, Nwadimma Uzoukwu, and Eric Christensen, *Military Medical Executive Education Review*, Alexandria, Va.: CNA Corporation, 2007.

Calhoun, Judith G., Lorayne Dollett, Marie E. Sinioris, Peter W. Butler, John R. Griffith, and Gail L. Warden, "Development of an Interprofessional Competency Model for Healthcare Leadership," *Journal of Healthcare Management*, Vol. 53, No. 6, November–December 2008, pp. 375–391.

Comarow, Avery, "What It Takes to Be the Best," *U.S. News and World Report*, July 15, 2007. As of May 26, 2010:
http://health.usnews.com/usnews/health/articles/070715/23meth.htm

Day, David V., and Stanley M. Halpin, *Leadership Development: A Review of Industry Best Practices*, Alexandria, Va.: U.S. Army Research Institute for the Behavioral and Social Sciences, 2001.

DoD—*see* U.S. Department of Defense.

DoDI—*see* U.S. Department of Defense Instruction.

Feeley, William F., Deputy Under Secretary for Health for Operations and Management, U.S. Department of Veterans Affairs, statement before the Subcommittee on Oversight and Investigations, Committee on Veterans' Affairs, U.S. House of Representatives, April 19, 2007. As of May 26, 2010: http://www4.va.gov/OCA/testimony/hvac/soi/070419WF.asp.

Garman, Andrew N., and J. Larry Tyler, *Succession Planning Practices and Outcomes in U.S. Hospital Systems: Final Report*, Prepared for the American College of Healthcare Executives, August 20, 2007.

Garvin, David A., Amy C. Edmondson, and Francesca Gino, "Is Yours a Learning Organization?" *Harvard Business Review*, March 2008, pp. 109–116.

HCA—*see* Hospital Corporation of America.

Headquarters, U.S. Department of the Army, *Army Medical Department Officer Development and Career Management*, Pamphlet 600-4, June 27, 2007.

———, *Commissioned Officer Professional Development and Career Management*, Pamphlet 600-3, February 1, 2010.

Healthcare Leadership Alliance, homepage, undated. As of May 26, 2010: http://www.healthcareleadershipalliance.org/

———, *HLA Competency Directory User's Guide*, Washington, D.C., November 2005. As of May 26, 2010: http://www.healthcareleadershipalliance.org/HLA_Competency_Directory_Guide.pdf

HLA—*see* Healthcare Leadership Alliance.

Hospital Corporation of America, "HCA Fact Sheet," undated. As of May 26, 2010: http://www.hcahealthcare.com/CPM/CurrentFactSheet1.pdf

Ibrahim, Said, "The Veterans Health Administration: A Domestic Model for a National Health Care System?" *American Journal of Public Health*, Vol. 97, No. 12, December 2007, pp. 2124–2126.

Jha, Ashish K., Jonathan B. Perlin, Kenneth W. Kizer, and R. Adams Dudley, "Effect of the Transformation of the Veterans Affairs Health Care System on Quality of Care," *New England Journal of Medicine*, Vol. 348, No. 22, May 29, 2003, pp. 2218–2227.

JMESI—*see* Joint Medical Executive Skills Institute.

Joint Medical Executive Skills Institute, homepage, undated. As of May 26, 2010: https://jmesi.army.mil/

———, Joint Medical Executive Skills Program: Core Curriculum, 6th ed., Ft. Sam Houston, Tex., September 2008.

Kaiser Permanente, "Fast Facts About Kaiser Permanente," web page, undated. As of May 26, 2010: http://xnet.kp.org/newscenter/aboutkp/fastfacts.html

Kerr, Eve A., and Barbara Fleming, "Making Performance Indicators Work: Experiences of US Veterans Health Administration," *British Medical Journal*, Vol. 335, No. 7627, November 10, 2007, pp. 971–973.

Kirby, Sheila Nataraj, and Harry J. Thie, *Qualifying Military Health Care Officers as "Joint": Weighing the Pros and Cons*, Santa Monica, Calif.: RAND Corporation, MG-775-OSD, 2009. As of May 26, 2010:
http://www.rand.org/pubs/monographs/MG775/

Kirkpatrick, Donald L., "Techniques for Evaluating Training Programs," *Journal for the American Society for Training and Development*, Vol. 13, No. 11, 1959, pp. 3–9.

———, *Evaluating Training Programs: The Four Levels*, San Francisco, Calif.: Berrett-Koehler, 1994.

Kizer, Kenneth W., *Vision for Change: A Plan to Restructure the Veterans Health Administration*, Washington, D.C.: Office of the Under Secretary for Health, U.S. Department of Veterans Affairs, March 17, 1995.

———, *Prescription for Change: The Guiding Principles and Strategic Objectives Underlying the Transformation of the Veterans Healthcare System*, Washington, D.C.: Office of the Under Secretary for Health, U.S. Department of Veterans Affairs, March 1996.

Marcus, Leonard J., Barry C. Dorn, and Joseph M. Henderson, *Meta-Leadership and National Emergency Preparedness: Strategies to Build Government Capacity*, Boston, Mass.: Center for Public Leadership, Harvard University, 2005. As of June 29, 2010:
http://www.hks.harvard.edu/leadership/Pdf/MarcusDornHendersonWorkingPaper.pdf

McAlearney, Ann Scheck, "Leadership Development in Healthcare: A Qualitative Study," *Journal of Organizational Behavior*, Vol. 27, No. 7, November 2006, pp. 967–982.

MHS—*see* Military Health System.

Military Health System, *Quadrennial Defense Review Roadmap for Medical Transformation*, April 3, 2006.

———, *Military Health System Strategic Plan*, Washington, D.C., April 2007a.

———, *MHS Human Capital Strategic Plan, 2008–2013*, Washington, D.C., November 2007b.

———, *Military Health System Strategic Plan: A Roadmap for Medical Transformation*, Summer 2008. As of May 26, 2010:
http://www.health.mil/Libraries/Documents_Word_PDF_PPT_etc/2008_Strat_Plan_Final_-lowres.pdf

National Center for Healthcare Leadership, "Leadership Excellence Networks™ (LENS)," web page, undated. As of May 26, 2010:
http://www.nchl.org/static.asp?path=2854,3212

———, "Henry Ford Health System Leadership," *NCHL Leadership Excellence Networks Executive Dialogue*, Vol. 1, No. 3, November 2006.

———, "Trinity Health Leadership," *NCHL Leadership Excellence Networks Executive Dialogue*, Vol. 3, No. 1, July 2008.

Oliver, Adam, "Public-Sector Health-Care Reforms That Work? A Case Study of the US Veterans Health Administration," *The Lancet*, Vol. 371, No. 9619, April 5, 2008, pp. 1211–1213.

Perlin, Jonathan B., Robert M. Kolodner, and Robert H. Roswell, "The Veterans Health Administration: Quality, Value, Accountability, and Information as Transforming Strategies for Patient-Centered Care," *American Journal of Managed Care*, Vol. 10, No. 11, November 2004, pp. 828–836.

Phillips, Jack J., ed., *Measuring Return on Investment*, Vol. 1, Alexandria, Va.: American Society for Training and Development, 1994.

Public Law 100-527, Department of Veterans Affairs Act, March 15, 1989.

Robbert, Albert, "Developing Leadership: Emulating the Military Model," in Robert Klitgaard and Paul C. Light, eds., *High-Performance Government: Structure, Leadership, Incentives*, Santa Monica, Calif.: RAND Corporation, MG-256-PRGS, 2005, pp. 255–280. As of May 26, 2010: http://www.rand.org/pubs/monographs/MG256/

Stoller, J. K., E. Berkowitz, and P. L. Bailin, "Physician Management and Leadership Education at the Cleveland Clinic Foundation: Program Impact and Experience Over 14 Years," *Journal of Medical Practice Management*, Vol. 22, No. 4, January–February 2007, pp. 237–242.

Thomson Reuters, "About the Top 100 Hospitals Program," web page, undated. As of May 26, 2010: http://www.100tophospitals.com/about-100-top-hospitals/

U.S. Army Medical Department, "Life Cycle Training Charts," web page, undated. As of May 26, 2010: http://www.cs.amedd.army.mil/lifecycle.aspx

———, "Levels of Care/Command and Control," web page, last modified July 8, 2008. As of May 26, 2010: http://www.armymedicine.army.mil/hc/medfacilities/CommandControl.htm

———, "Army Medicine Mission Statement," web page, last modified May 26, 2010. As of May 26, 2010: http://www.armymedicine.army.mil/about/mission.html

U.S. Department of Defense, *Capstone Concept for Joint Operations*, version 2.0, Washington, D.C., August 2005. As of May 26, 2010: http://www.dtic.mil/futurejointwarfare/concepts/approved_ccjov2.pdf

———, *Quadrennial Defense Review Report*, Washington, D.C., February 6, 2006. As of May 26, 2010: http://www.defense.gov/qdr/report/Report20060203.pdf

———, *Joint Officer Management: Joint Qualification System Implementation Plan*, Washington, D.C., March 30, 2007.

———, *Report of the Tenth Quadrennial Review of Military Compensation*, Vol. 1, *Cash Compensation*, Washington, D.C., February 2008a. As of May 26, 2010: http://www.whs.mil/library/doc/Tenth.pdf

———, *Report of the Tenth Quadrennial Review of Military Compensation*, Vol. 2, *Deferred and Noncash Compensation*, Washington, D.C., July 2008b. As of May 26, 2010: http://www.defense.gov/news/QRMCreport.pdf

U.S. Department of Defense Directive 1020.02, Diversity Management and Equal Opportunity (EO) in the Department of Defense, February 5, 2009.

——— 3000.5, Military Support for Stability, Security, Transition, and Reconstruction (SSTR) Operations, November 28, 2005.

——— 6000.12, Health Services Operations and Readiness, April 29, 1996, incorporating change 1, January 20, 1998, certified current as of November 24, 2003.

U.S. Department of Defense Instruction 1300.19, DoD Joint Officer Management Program, October 31, 2007, incorporating change 2, February 16, 2010.

——— 1300.20, Joint Officer Management Program Procedures, December 20, 1996.

———— 6000.13, Medical Manpower and Personnel, June 30, 1997.

U.S. Department of the Navy, Bureau of Medicine and Surgery, "Navy Nurse Corps Planning Chart (01-06)," Washington, D.C., June 2005.

U.S. Department of Veterans Affairs, "High Performance Development Model (HPDM): Core Competency Definitions and Behavioral Examples at Each Level," undated.

————, Veterans Health Administration, "Developing Leaders at All Levels," brochure, September 1, 2007a.

————, *Veterans Health Administration Workforce Succession Strategic Plan, FY 2008–2012*, Washington, D.C., October 2007b.

————, *High Performance Development Model Pocket Guide, Level 4*, Washington, D.C., 2008a.

————, *FY 2008 VHA Executive Career Field Performance Plan—Final*, updated February 21, 2008b.

————, *Veterans Health Administration Workforce Succession Strategic Plan*, Washington, D.C., 2009a.

————, *Department of Veterans Affairs Organizational Briefing Book*, Washington, D.C., June 2009b. As of May 26, 2010:
http://www4.va.gov/ofcadmin/docs/vaorgbb.pdf

————, "PBI Site," web page (click "PBI Links" for full selection of resources), last updated May 28, 2010. As of June 2, 2010:
http://www4.va.gov/pbi/

U.S. Joint Chiefs of Staff, *CJCS Vision for Joint Officer Development*, Washington, D.C., November 2005. As of May 26, 2010:
https://acc.dau.mil/CommunityBrowser.aspx?id=250129